D1384343

Antihypertensive Agents

Edward L. Engelhardt, EDITOR

*Merck Sharp & Dohme
Research Laboratories*

A symposium sponsored by

the Division of Medicinal

Chemistry at the 169th

Meeting of the American

Chemical Society,

Philadelphia, Penn.,

April 8, 1975

A C S   S Y M P O S I U M   S E R I E S   **27**

AMERICAN CHEMICAL SOCIETY

WASHINGTON, D. C.   1976

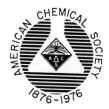

Library of Congress CIP Data

Antihypertensive agents.
  (ACS symposium series; 27 ISSN 0097-6156)

  Includes bibliographical references and index.

  1. Hypotensive agents—Congresses. 2. Adrenergic beta
receptor blockaders—Congresses.
  I. Engelhardt, Edward L., 1919-   . II. American
Chemical Society. Division of Medicinal Chemistry. III.
Series: American Chemical Society. ACS symposium se-
ries; 27. [DNLM: 1. Antihypertensive agents—Congresses.
2. Hypertension—Drug therapy—Congresses.   WG340
A629 1975].

RM345.A57   615'.71   76-15416
ISBN 0-8412-0333-4   ACSMC8 27 1–96

ACS Symposium Series

Robert F. Gould, *Series Editor*

FOREWORD

The ACS SYMPOSIUM SERIES was founded in 1974 to provide
a medium for publishing symposia quickly in book form. The
format of the SERIES parallels that of the continuing ADVANCES
IN CHEMISTRY SERIES except that in order to save time the
papers are not typeset but are reproduced as they are sub-
mitted by the authors in camera-ready form. As a further
means of saving time, the papers are not edited or reviewed
except by the symposium chairman, who becomes editor of
the book. Papers published in the ACS SYMPOSIUM SERIES
are original contributions not published elsewhere in whole or
major part and include reports of research as well as reviews
since symposia may embrace both types of presentation.

CONTENTS

PREFACE

During the quarter of a century that I have been involved in the search for antihypertensive agents, there has been a continuing trend by the clinician to use antihypertensive therapy in patients with less and less severe hypertensive disease. This has led to a need for agents that are effective in milder degrees of hypertension and substantially free from side effects that might reduce compliance of the patient with the therapeutic regimen.

The four papers that comprise this volume provide a concise overview of the current status of antihypertensive agents in use or in the later stages of development in 1975. The saluretic diuretics are not described in detail, although G. Onesti discusses their importance as an integral part of the antihypertensive therapeutic armamentarium. The intensive and extensive research in β-adrenergic blocking agents is critically reviewed by R. Clarkson. W. Hoefke discusses the centrally acting antihypertensive agents as typified by clonidine and methyldopa. J. E. Francis presents a comprehensive survey of antihypertensive agents with peripheral sites of action. Finally, Onesti discusses the clinician's use of various antihypertensive agents in providing optimal therapy.

The development of new agents to permit better control of blood pressure while restoring normal hemodynamics with minimal side effects presents a continuing challenge to the medicinal chemist. Doubtless improved agents that fall into the pharmacological classes now recognized will be developed. The complexity of the interplay of neural and renal factors involved in the control of blood pressure gives hope that other points for therapeutic intervention will be found as our basic knowledge of the pathophysiology of hypertensive vascular disease increases.

Merck Sharp & Dohme   EDWARD L. ENGELHARDT
Research Laboratories
West Point, Pa.
December 22, 1975

β-Adrenoceptor Antagonists as Antihypertensive Agents

RICHARD CLARKSON

Imperial Chemical Industries Ltd., Pharmaceuticals Division,
Hurdsfield Industrial Estate, Macclesfield Chesire, England.

The search for specific β-adrenoceptor antagonists was initiated in the belief that protection of the ischaemic, myocardium from adrenergic stimulation would be clinically valuable in the treatment of angina pectoris and post-infarct patients. Clinical studies with the early compounds (especially propranolol) not only confirmed the belief but showed the agents to have several other therapeutic uses (1) perhaps the most significant of which is their anti-hypertensive action. This action was first discovered by Prichard in 1964 (2) using propranolol. The hypotensive effect of a β-blocking agent was so totally unexpected that some scepticism surrounded the observation particularly as it seemed that enormous doses were generally required (relative to those required for complete β-blockade) and that even then, the falls in blood pressure were only modest. However, the large number of subsequent investigations have adequately confirmed Pritchard's findings (except perhaps for the necessity of the massive doses - see later), have shown that the anti-hypertensive effect is a property of β-blocking agents as a class, and have established these drugs as possibly the treatment of choice for essential hypertension.(3)

Despite intensive research the precise mechanism by which β-blocking drugs lower blood pressure in clinical use is still uncertain although several fascinating hypotheses have been advanced and some partly validated by experiment.

One major difficulty has been that no convincing laboratory model of the drug's clinical effect has yet been established. This has not only hampered mechanistic investigations but has also prevented the rational search, by medicinal chemists, for more specifically effective anti-hypertensive β-blocking agents. New drug candidates appear to have been selected on the basis of the laboratory pharmacological profile of the molecule and how this profile relates to one or other of the various mode-of-action hypotheses.

The medicinal chemist expects to find that a review written specifically for him will be mainly concerned with a discussion of structure/activity relationships. In the case of the anti-hypertensive activity of the β-blockers such a discussion is not possible since no direct comparative activity data is available either from the laboratory or the clinic (the few comparative clinical studies are in no way definitive - see later). It is however possible to approach the problem somewhat indirectly and consider the influence of chemical structure on those pharmacological properties which appear most relevant to the specific clinical effect. I propose therefore to:-

1)   outline some correlations of chemical structure with some of the standard pharmacological properties of the series;

2)   compare the laboratory pharmacological profiles and clinical comparative appraisals of the hypotensive effect of a representative section of the β-blocking drugs;

3)   consider the characteristics of the hypotensive response in relation to some mode-of-action hypotheses; and

4)   summarise the available evidence in terms of suggestions about the properties required for an anti-hypertensive β-blocking drug.

This review is not intended to be exhaustive. Its aim is to provide an insight into the problems and questions surrounding the study of the hypotensive activity of the β-adrenergic antagonists and to illustrate possible avenues along which answers may be, and are being sought. Most of the data quoted is from our own laboratory and many of the ideas and views expressed are those currently held by chemists, clinicians and biologists from this laboratory.

Before moving into a discussion of chemical structure and pharmacological properties of the β-blocking molecules, may we briefly consider some of the key points in the discovery and development of the series as a whole.

By ranking the sensitivity of a range of sympathetically innervated tissues to a number of sympathomimetic amines Ahlquist (4) proposed that the tissues contained two types of receptor and labelled them α and β. The tissues served predominantly by β-adrenergic receptors (β-adrenoceptors) are shown in figure 1. Lands (5) later suggested a sub-division of the β-adrenoceptors and classified those serving heart and adipose tissue as β_1 and those serving bronchi and blood vessels as β_2. Thus a β_1-adrenoceptor stimulant produces an increase in cardiac rate, force of contraction and conduction velocity together with an increase in lypolysis; while a β_2-adrenoceptor stimulant causes bronchial relaxation and dilatation of the blood vessels in certain vascular beds (e.g. skeletal muscle).

The natural sympathetic transmitter substance (i.e. that released at terminals following sympathetic nerve stimulation) is noradrenaline figure 2. When administered

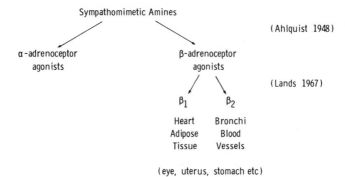

Figure 1.   *The Ahlquist–Lands classification of the sympmathomi-
metic amines*

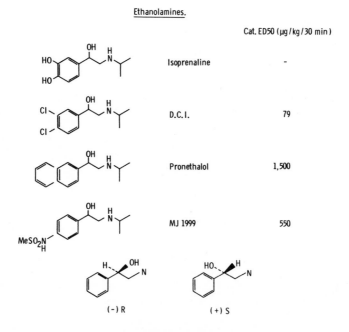

Figure 2.   *Isoprenaline and the early ethanolamine β-adrenergic
antagonists*

systemically to animals its predominant effect is α-stimulation.
The N-isopropyl analogue, isoprenaline, on the other hand shows
predominantly a β-effect and has become the standard stimulus
against which antagonists are tested.

Dichloro-isoprenaline was the first β-adrenoceptor
antagonist to be described (6). It was discovered in a search
for specific β-stimulants as bronchodilators. This compound
is a partial agonist, i.e. it can antagonise the action of
isoprenaline but itself is a β-stimulant. (The stimulant action
of dichloro-isoprenaline is readily demonstrated in an animal
depleted of natural catecholamines (with say reserpine). In
this type of preparation it will stimulate say heart rate to a
maximum of 70% of that produced by isoprenaline itself).
β-Blocking agents which can also stimulate the β-receptor are
said to show intrinsic sympathomimetic activity (i.s.a.). The
very high level of i.s.a. shown by dichloro-isoprenaline was
thought by Black and Stevenson to be undesirable in a compound
designed to protect the ischaemic myocardium from sympathetic
drive. They thus began their search for a compound showing
much less i.s.a. and of course discovered pronethalol (7) the
first β-blocking drug to be tested in man. The success of this
work has led to the tremendous, almost explosive expansion of
research in this field (8).

Structure/activity relationships among these, the
ethanolamine series of β-blockers,(i.e. as illustrated by
pronethalol and sotalol, MJ1999) have been extensively reviewed
(8,9.) One general point which needs to be emphasised is that
the structure/activity pattern with respect to modifications of
the ethanolamine side-chain closely parallels that found for
the β-stimulants, particularly with respect to type of amino-
substituent required. Another point is that both blocking and
stimulant activity lie with the R-enantiomer.

Modifying the way in which the aromatic system was linked
to the ethanolamine moiety led to the oxypropranolamines as
typified by propranolol. It is 10-20 times more potent than
pronethalol and shows no intrinsic sympathomimetic activity.
The success of propranolol stimulated intense synthetic activity
in many laboratories. Several thousand oxypropanolamine
analogues were produced, of these 30 - 40 have been studied in
man and some 14 are commercially available.

Three examples are given in figure 3.

Structure Activity Relationships

May we now consider the four pharmacological properties of
the β-blockers most commonly studied in the laboratory and at the
same time review the highlights of the structural correlations
of the oxypropranolamines with each action.

(1) Cardiac β-adrenergic blocking potency. This is obviously

the key pharmacological property of the molecules – its presence
defines the series. There are now several standard tests for
measuring cardiac β-blocking potency both <u>in vivo</u> and <u>in vitro</u>
which depend on measuring the antagonism by the test compound
of the cardiac action of the β-stimulant isoprenaline. Our
laboratory screen test is against a standard isoprenaline induced
tachycardia in the anaesthetised cat and activity is recorded as
the dose ($\mu g/kg/$infused i.v. over 30 min.) to produce a 50% block.
(This is termed ED_{50} and except where stated, all references to
potency in this review are based on this test).

Within the phenoxypropanolamines, what are the basic
structural requirements for cardiac β-blocking activity? Simply
an appropriately substituted aminopropanol moiety linked through
an ether oxygen to an aromatic system. Within these basic
requirements there is enormous scope for structural variety.
This fact, coupled with the easy synthesis of the molecule has
meant that vast numbers have been prepared and tested (<u>8</u>). The
effect of structural change on β-blocking activity is most
conveniently examined if we divide the structural modifications
into two kinds. Firstly, there are those which directly modify
the parts of the molecule that are clearly involved in bonding
to the receptors. These effects of structural change are
<u>specific</u> and in general have an all-or-none influence on activity
and thus can not be correlated. Secondly there are those
modifications which produce <u>non-specific</u> effects changing say
the total lipophylicity or charge density. Their effects can
clearly be correlated in some fashion. Hopefully an examination
of the biological activity of any series of molecules permits
one to identify most of the areas of structural changes which
produce specific effects and thus simplify the total structure/
activity picture by a suitable correlation of the remaining
non-specific effects. To a certain extent this has been
achieved with the phenoxypropanolamine β-blocking drugs.

Consider first the oxypropanolamine side chain <u>figure 4.</u>
Substitution on the α-,β or γ carbon atoms markedly lowers
activity. Methylation of the hydroxyl group renders the molecule
inactive – the corresponding acetate is still active but probably
through being hydrolysed to the free hydroxyl group. In general
the effects of variations on the side chain closely parallel
those found for both the ethanolamine β-agonists and the antagonists. This was particularly true of N-substitution – the
isopropyl and t-butyl groups usually being preferred. (Although
recently more complex side chains have been used – <u>cf</u> tolamolol
(<u>11</u>) later). The absolute configuration of the hydroxyl group is
also the same in both series. (N.B. although the "active"
ethanolamines have the "R" configuration and the propanolamines
the "S", they have in fact the same absolute configuration). The
groups on the side chain are clearly involved in bonding to the
receptor and the effects of structural change are <u>specific</u>.

Turning now to the effects of substitution in the phenyl ring

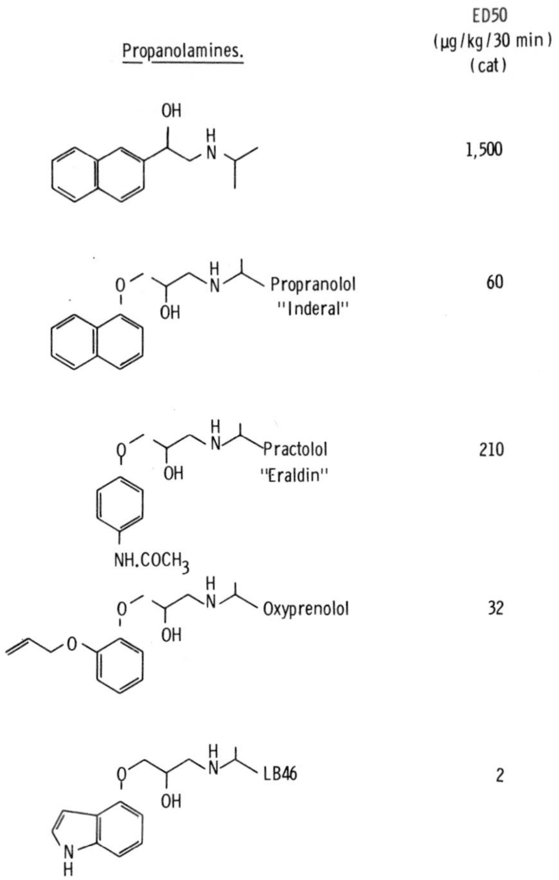

Figure 3. Some β-blocking agents of the propanolamine series

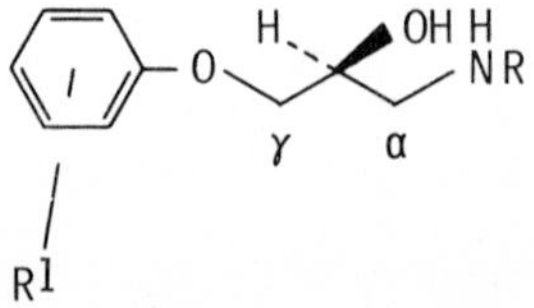

S - configuration

Figure 4. Cardiac β-blocking activity of the aryloxypropanolamines—modification of the side-chain

we can see, by a consideration of the β-blocking activity of
pairs of <u>ortho</u> and <u>para</u> substituted analogues <u>figure 5</u> that both
<u>specific</u> and <u>non-specific</u> effects are involved.

The compounds are arranged so that the substituents fall
into 3 groups. The first group contains essentially non-
interacting substituents - note that the <u>ortho</u>-substituted
compound is more active than the <u>para</u> and that the difference
appears greater, the larger the group. In the second group the
substituent is attached to the aromatic ring through a trigonal
carbon - here the <u>ortho</u>, <u>para</u> difference is even more startling.
In the final group the substituent bears an exchangeable
hydrogen - the above trend is now reversed and the <u>para</u>-
substituent becomes the more active.

Our interpretation of the results was that the <u>para</u>-
substituent was involved in a specific interaction (we define
this more clearly later) with the receptor. We then found (this
is the work of Dr R. H. Davies) that if we divided our β-blockers
into classes according to the type of <u>para</u>-substituent, we were
then able to do a Hansch type regression (<u>12</u>) (using π and σ) on
each class and get quite meaningful results.

As an example I would like to consider the <u>para</u>-acylamino
"class" of propanolamines as developed from practolol. These
have the general formula:-

where R_1 = tBu or iPr

Some 150 compounds were considered and the best fit
regression equation devised using π values for the total molecule
and σ_m values for the <u>ortho</u>-substituent R_2, together with two all-
or-nothing-terms to handle two minor specific effects.

$$\mathrm{Log}\left(\frac{ED50 \times 100}{M.Wt}\right) = 2.21 - 0.80\pi + 0.128\pi^2 - 1.16\sigma_{m_1} - 0.275\sigma_{m_2}$$
$$-0.30\delta_{R_1} + 0.30\delta_{R_3}$$

(r=0.980; r.s.d.= ± 0.141; mean experimental error=± 0.12)

based on Practolol-R_1 = iPr; R_2 = H, R_3 = Me

where σ_{m_1} and σ_{m_2} are the meta-electronic effects of R_2 and

$$\text{when } R_1 = tBu, \; \sigma_{m_2} = 0$$
$$\text{when } R_1 = iPr, \; \sigma_{m_1} = 0$$
$$\text{when } R_1 = iPr, \; \delta_{R_1} = 0$$
$$\text{when } R_1 = tBu, \; \delta_{R_1} = 1$$
$$\text{when } R_3 = Me \text{ or } Et, \; \delta_{R_3} = 0$$
$$\text{when } R_3 = \; \ngtr nPr, \; \delta_{R_3} = 1$$

The conclusions derived from this equation are illustrated diagramatically in figure 6 and may be summarised as follows:-

(i)   Increasing lipophilicity increased activity.

(ii)   The ortho portion was relatively sterically free and could tolerate quite large groups without them causing a significant fall in activity.

(iii)   Electron withdrawing substituents in the ortho position increased activity. The correlation was with the Hammett σ_m value and was interpreted as increasing the acidity of the para-amidic NH proton and hence strengthening a hydrogen bond to an acceptor site on the receptor (designated C=O). (A para substituent unable to make such a hydrogen bond would sterically hinder the acceptor site and hence would give a less active molecule). In other amidic "classes" where the NH is not directly attached to the aromatic ring (such as the para - benzamides) the electronic influence of the ortho-substituent weakens. When R_1 is tBu the electronic influence of the ortho- substituent is enhanced.

(iv)   There was a step-drop in activity as the R group of the acyl residue was lengthened from ethyl to n-propyl. There was no further drop on extending this chain further. This presumably indicates a kind of "steric-narrows" at a distance of 4 to 5 atoms from the 4-position of the aromatic ring when the molecule is attached to the receptor. A similar step-drop was seen with other classes as the para-side chain was lengthened through this critical distance.

(v)   t-Butyl analogues were more active than were i-propyl analogues.

From the basic information derived for the para-acylamino class, we were able to derive regression equations for other classes using the first few examples synthesised and to use these to predict (in some cases with remarkable accuracy) the ED_{50} values for further compounds of that class. One example, the para-urieido-series is illustrated by the results given in table 1.

The regression equation was derived from the first ten examples of the para-ureido class and used to predict the next dozen made. In 5 cases the prediction was out by a factor of 2 in the other 7 it was well within a two fold variation. Considering that the compounds span a twenty fold range of activity, the calculated ED_{50} values are extremely close to the

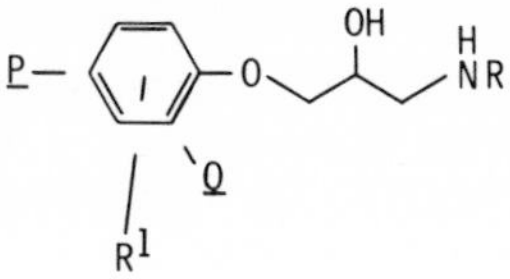

$$\underline{P}-\underset{\underset{R^1}{|}}{\overset{I}{\bigcirc}}-O-\underset{\underset{OH}{|}}{CH}-CH_2-\overset{H}{N}R$$

R^1	R	$\underline{O}$-ED50	$\underline{p}$-ED50
Me	Bu^t	20	600
Cl	Bu^t	68	276
Ph	Pr^i	75	1,000
F	Pr^i	26	50
H | C=O	Pr^i	17	NA
CH$_3$ | C=O	Bu^t	4	3,818
H | C=N.N=CH—$\boxed{_S}$	Bu^t	16	NA
NH.SO$_2$Me	Pr^i	300	160
NH.CO.CH$_3$	Pr^i	480	210
NH.CO.NH.Et	Bu^t	NA	200
OH	Pr^i	150	25

Figure 5. Cardiac β-blocking activity of the aryloxypropanolamines—effect of ortho and para-substitution in the aromatic ring

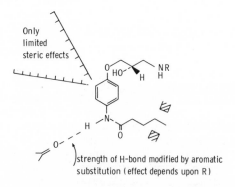

Figure 6. Cardiac β-blocking activity of the aryloxypropanolamines—summary of specific effects

experimental ones.

However, although the accuracy of these predictions is impressive one must remember that they apply to a very closely defined series. We are still unable to predict the specific effects of substituents and have no answer to the intriguing question of why does the introduction of the OCH_2 unit into the phenylethanolamines give such good β-blockers, or why the addition of a polar group (amide or ether) to a para-alkyl substituent to some extent relieves the steric crowding (cf ICI 66082 (13) and metoprolol (14)) table 2.

Table 1 - The para-Ureido Series

$$R_3NHCONH - \underset{R2}{\bigcirc} - O \underset{OH}{\longrightarrow} \overset{H}{NR_1}$$

R_1	R_2	R_3	ED50 (μg/kg) predicted	ED50 (μg/kg) observed
$CH(CH_3)_2$	Br	CH_3	31	30
"	CH_3	CH_3	98	174
"	Cl	CH_3	44	92
$C(CH_3)_3$	Cl	CH_3	9	17.4
$CH(CH_3)_2$	Br	C_2H_5	67	69
$CH(CH_3)_2$	Cl	C_2H_5	90	186
$C(CH_3)_3$	I	C_2H_5	24	22
$CH(CH_3)_2$	H	C_3H_7	110	135
$CH(CH_3)_2$	H	$CH(CH_3)_2$	110	93
$C(CH_3)_3$	CH_3	C_3H_7	47	45
$CH(CH_3)_2$	CH_3	C_4H_9	72	49
$C(CH_3)_3$	Cl	C_4H_9	7.0	8.4

(2) Intrinsic Sympathomimetic Activity. The majority of β-blocking molecules are partial agonists showing varying amounts of i.s.a. It is in fact quite difficult to design a pure non-stimulant β-blocker such as propranolol. Measurement of i.s.a. has to be done using an animal depleted of catechol-amines. Our own laboratory test measures the increase in heart rate (bts./min) when a single high dose (2.5 mg/kg iv.) is given to a rat depleted of natural catecholamines by prior administration of syrosingopine.

Structural requirements for i.s.a. among the β-blocking molecules are far from clear though an inspection of some of the data available permits certain generalisations to be made.

Considering first the series of phenoxypropanolamines illustrated in Table 2 we can see that although the unsubstituted phenoxy analogue shows a high level of i.s.a. this is rapidly diminished as the size of the ortho-substituent is increased. Introducing electronegative substituents into the para-position (giving practolol and H 87/07) produces compounds still retaining high levels of i.s.a. However if one interposes methylene groups between the electronegative groups and the aromatic ring (giving metoprolol and ICI 66082) i.s.a. is virtually eliminated. Another example of a molecular change resulting in a sharp drop in i.s.a. is illustrated by comparing tolamolol with the second molecule in the table. We see that the change is the replacement of the N-isopropyl substituent by an N-aryloxyethyl residue.

Table 2 – Effect of Aryloxy Group on i.s.a. (1)

Phenoxy analogues

Compound	X	i.s.a.*	R
	H	104 ± 7	iPr
	o–Me	65 ± 7	"
	o–Et	29 ± 7	"
H 87/07	p–MeO(CH$_2$)O	(>practolol)	"
practolol	p–AcNH	78	"
metoprolol	p–MeO(CH$_2$)$_2$	(0)	"
ICI 66082	p–H$_2$NCOCH$_2$	0	"
tolamolol	o–Me	(0)	(CH$_2$)$_2$O C$_6$H$_4$CONH$_2$

(*tachycardia in beats/min following 2.5 mg/kg i.v. to syrosingopinised rat)

Several interesting effects of structural change on i.s.a. are illustrated by the compounds shown in Figure 7. (The figures show the level of i.s.a. as defined above). To the left are shown the aromatic moieties of propranolol, pindolol (LB 46) and

timolol. The striking effect on the i.s.a. of substituting the
indole residue of pindolol for the naphthalene group of
propranolol is obvious and one is tempted to postulate that the
indole NH group is perhaps beginning to take on the role of the
catechol group of the full agonists. That the thiadiazole
timolol shows no i.s.a. is not surprising in view of its bulky
ortho-substituent.

The three compounds on the right of Figure 7 show the effect
of conformation on i.s.a. Linking the methoxy group to the
1-position of the side chain results in a lowering of i.s.a.
while linking it to the 2-position produces a marked increase.
In fact the benzdioxepine is more of a stimulant than a blocker.
In the syrosingopinised rat test a full agonist such as
isoprenaline only produces an increase in heart rate of 200-210
beats/min.

A tentative correlation between the population of specific
conformers about the 1, 2-carbon-carbon bond and i.s.a. has
emerged in a preliminary molecular orbital study on a series of
ortho-substituted phenoxypropanolamines (15)

(3) Cardioselectivity. The data from which Lands postulated the
sub-division of β-receptors (5) together with that derived from
the research into β_2-specific agonists as bronchodilators (16),
imply that the β_1 and β_2 types of receptor are chemically
different. The finding (17) that, para-substitution tended to
give cardioselective blockers while ortho-substitution gave non-
selective agents also lends support to this view. The results
from our laboratory however, suggest that the cardiac and
pulmonary β-receptors are identical with respect to the interaction of β-blocking molecules, and that tissue selectivity
results from differences in non-specific interactions and is in
effect due to differences in distribution of the molecules to the
micro-environment surrounding the receptor*. An attempt to
graphically illustrate these results is shown in Figure 8.

The effectiveness as a β-blocker of any particular molecule
(i.e. its ED_{50}) may be considered as two terms: the first is the
energy of binding to the receptor and the second is a term
representing the molecule's distribution to the receptor site.
The distributive term is essentially related to the partition
coefficient thus if we subtract this distributive term from the
ED_{50} we arrive at an estimate of the binding energy of the
molecule at the receptor site. We refer to this binding energy
as intrinsic β-blocking activity or i.b.a. thus:-

$$i.b.a. = \log\left(\frac{ED_{50} \times 100}{M.Wt}\right) - A\pi + B\pi^2$$

*This is the work of Dr. R. H. Davies of ICI Pharmaceuticals
 Division whose permission to publish is gratefully acknowledged.

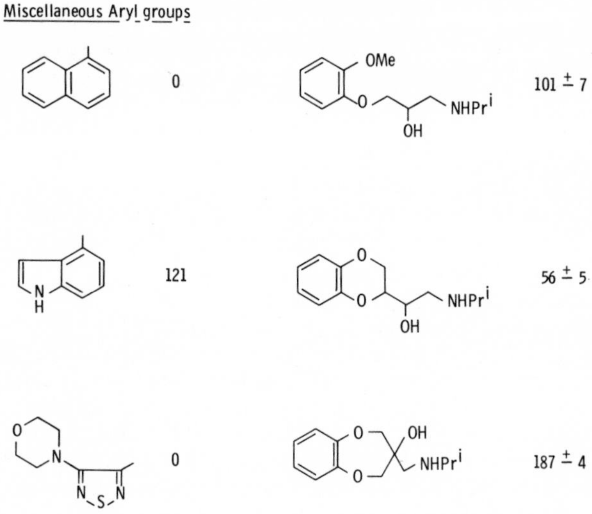

Miscellaneous Aryl groups

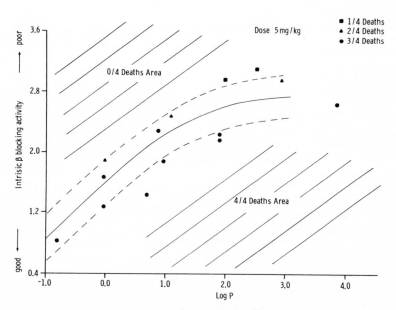

British Medical Journal

Figure 7.   Effect of aryloxy group on i.s.a. (2)

Figure 8.   Relation between receptor binding affinity, lipid character, and isoprenaline antagonism in the guinea pig bronchospasm test

where A and B are constants derived from the regression equation
for the particular series in question. Plotting this against log
P gives a family of parallel isopotency lines (for the cardiac
site) one of which is shown in Figure 8.

The actual shape of the isopotency curves identifies the
binding characteristics of the particular receptor site (in this
case the cardiac site). If a plot of i.b.a.'s derived from
pulmonary ED_{50} data provided a family of different shaped curves
then one could safely conclude that the cardiac and pulmonary
β-receptors were indeed different.

However a series of pulmonary ED_{50}'s were not available to
us since our standard screen test for bronchial β-blockade
measures the inhibitory effect of a single fixed dose on the
protective action of isoprenaline against histamine induced
bronchospasm in the guinea pig. Groups of four animals are used
and the results are expressed as numbers of animals dead within
the group. However simply identifying, on the cardiac i.b.a.
versus log P plot, those compounds which on the bronchospasm
test gave 1, 2 or 3 survivors (i.e. the dose used approximates
to the ED_{50}) would give a clear indication of whether the
bronchial isopotency curve would follow the cardiac one.
Figure 8 shows that it in fact does. (N.B. Although the
compounds cover a 300 fold range of i.b.a. they almost all fall
within a factor of two (cf. dotted lines) of the cardiac
isopotency line shown. Furthermore compounds showing 0/4 and a
4/4 deaths as expected, appeared in the areas shown).

Although this correlation uses rather crude data it gives a
clear indication that the actual antagonist/receptor binding is
the same at both the cardiac and bronchial sites and indicates
that cardioselectivity is a function of distribution to the
micro-environment of the receptor site. Some experimental
evidence supporting this conclusion is now available from
biochemical studies on isolated membrane fragments derived from
heart and lung*.

Table 3 shows pA_2 values for practolol and propranolol
against isoprenaline induced tachycardia in the guinea pig atria,
relaxation of the tracheal chain, and adenylate cyclase activity
of purified membrane fragments prepared from guinea pig heart
and lung. While practolol is clearly cardioselective in the
tissue preparations it becomes non-selective on the membrane
fragments. It is conceivable that in the purification of the
membranes the integrity of the micro-environment which controls
access to the receptors in the different tissues, is destroyed.

Our current belief is that cardioselectivity is more likely
to be found with those β-blocking molecules containing hydrogen
bond acceptor groups.

*Results of Dr. A. R. Somerville and Mr. A. J. Coleman of the
  Biochemistry Dept., ICI Pharmaceuticals Division whose
  permission to publish them here is gratefully acknowledged.

Table 3 - pA$_2$ Values for Practolol and Propranolol on Heart
and Lung Tissue and Membranes

		pA$_2$	
		Tissue	Membranes
propranolol	heart	8.32	8.57
	lung	7.60	8.61
practolol	heart	6.49	5.56
	lung	4.66	5.58

(pA$_2$ is the negative logarithm of the concentration of
antagonist which requires a doubling of the agonist
concentration to maintain the same level of response
from the tissue)

(4) Membrane Stabilising Activity (m.s.a.) Many of the
β-blocking molecules exhibit a range of pharmacological effects
all of which are due to a modification of the cell membrane
structure which results in a decrease of ion transport across the
membrane. The type of actions produced are non-specific cardiac
depression, depression of myocardial conduction velocity, local
anaesthetic activity, reversal of cardiac glycoside induced
arrhythmias, quinidine-like activity, depression of calcium ion
uptake in sarcoplasmic reticulum vesicles, etc.
      Hellenbrecht and co-workers (18) have now produced con-
clusive evidence showing that the magnitude of these membrane
effects correlate directly with lipophilicity.
      Many groups of workers still measure m.s.a. for new
β-blocking molecules and associate its absence with increased
safety. There is however overwhelming evidence to show that
these effects are without clinical significance (19). The main
reason for including this section in this review is that those
compounds showing m.s.a. are highly lipophilic and hence would
more readily concentrate in the central nervous system than
would the less lipophilic analogues showing no m.s.a. This will
be an important consideration when we come to discuss the
centrally mediated anti-hypertensive action of the β-blocking
molecules.

Anti-hypertensive Properties

      Having considered the general relationships of chemical
structure with these four different pharmacological actions,
might we first look in detail at six compounds whose clinical

anti-hypertensive properties have been compared to see if there
is any correlation between laboratory pharmacology and the anti-
hypertensive action in man. And secondly, may we move on to
consider the evidence for some of the more popular mode-of-
action hypotheses and try to relate these to the known pharmacology of the β-blockers (20).

(1) Comparative Studies. Table 4 shows the laboratory pharmacological profiles of these six β-blocking drugs. It will be
noted that the compounds have quite different profiles, (although
pindolol and alprenolol appear superficially similar, pindolol is
in fact far more potent as both an antagonist and as a stimulant)
potency varies over a 100 fold range, 4 of the 6 are partial
agonists, 2 are cardioselective and half show m.s.a.

Table 4. Typical Laboratory Pharmacological Profiles

	Relative potency (cardiac)	i.s.a.	m.s.a.	Cardioselectivity
propranolol	1.0	–	+	–
alprenolol	1.0	+	+	–
pindolol	30	+	+	–
timolol	10	–	–	–
practolol	0.3	+	–	+
ICI 66082	1.0	–	–	+

Although these six compounds have not been directly compared with each other sufficient clinical comparisons have been
made to permit one to assess the relative effectiveness of all
the compounds. The studies are listed in Table 5.

Table 5. Clinical Comparisons of β-blocking Drugs in Hypertension

propranolol vs. alprenolol	(Bengtsson 1972) (21) (Berglund & Hannson 1973) (22)
propranolol vs. timolol	(Franciosa et al. 1973) (23) (Lohmoller et al. 1972) (24)
propranolol vs. practolol	(Zacharias 1974) (25)
propranolol vs. ICI 66082	(Zacharias 1975) (26)
propranolol, timolol, pindolol, alprenolol	(Morgan et al. 1974) (27)

The most striking conclusion from these studies is that the hypotensive response is virtually the same for all six drugs. Although in some of the studies a statistically significant difference has been observed (e.g. in Zacharias' two studies, ICI 66082 was slightly more effective than propranolol which itself was slightly more effective than practolol) the difference is of little consequence clinically. The most detailed comparative study was that of Morgan et al in which no significant differences were found between any of the four drugs used.

There was however a marked difference between the doses required to produce the optimum hypotensive effect (as is shown in Table 6.)

Table 6. Anti-anginal and Anti-hypertensive Dose Compared to Experimental Cardiac β-blocking Potency

	Explt.Cardiac β-blocking potency	Anti-anginal dose mg/day	Anti-hypertensive dose mg/day
propranolol	1	60 - 240	240 - 480
alprenolol	1	150 - 400	400 - 800
pindolol	30	2.5 - 5	15 - 45
timolol	10	15 - 40	30 - 60
practolol	0.3	200 - 600	600 - 1,200
ICI 66082	1		100 - 200

The anti-hypertensive dose is clearly related to the dose used to treat angina although the former is a good deal higher than the latter. Both doses however clearly correlate with the experimental cardiac β-blocking potency.

There appears to be no relationship between the anti-hypertensive activity of the β-blocking agents and the other three laboratory pharmacological parameters.

One must therefore conclude from these comparisons that provided sufficient drug is given to maintain an effective blockade of the cardiac β-receptor, all β-blockers appear to produce equal falls in blood pressure.

(2) Mode-of-Action Hypotheses. May we now turn to consider some of the suggested mechanisms put forward to explain the hypotensive action of the β-blocking drugs and see if any are compatible with the clinical and pharmacological data. Before doing so however, it perhaps would be useful to summarise the characteristics of the anti-hypertensive action of the drugs.

These are:-

(i) Only 50-70% of patients respond - This can be
increased by adding a diuretic and/or a vasodilator to
the treatment. The 3-drug combination has been found
to control blood pressure in subjects previously
refractory to other forms of treatment (28).

(ii) The compounds do not have a dramatic effect on
blood pressure, i.e. in general falls of 20/12 mm.Hg
are observed although in some of the large open trials
the reduction appears more marked (e.g. 58/32 mm.Hg)
but probably contains some "placebo" effect (3).

(iii) There is a delay after dosing begins before
the onset of the hypotensive effect. Some confusion
still remains with respect to the time required for
the β-blocking drugs to achieve their full anti-
hypertensive effect. Earlier studies suggested that
the effect developed over several weeks or even months.
While more recent trials with the newer compounds
shows that a good effect may be achieved within 48
hours (see later). One possible explanation of this
discrepancy is that in the early studies the dosage
was slowly raised over a period while the current
practice is to use the full anti-hypertensive dose
from the outset (20). It may also be that the fall
in blood pressure occurs in two phases.
There is no doubt, however, that the anti-hypertensive
effect of the β-blocking drugs is not immediate - a
characteristic which one must take into consideration
in examining some of the proposed mechanisms of action.

(iv) Good control of blood pressure is achieved both
in the supine and upright positions. This is of course
of clear advantage over some forms of anti-hypertensive
therapy especially in the case of patients prone to
hypertensive complications.

(v) No postural hypotension.

(vi) Few side effects.

      Bearing these characteristics in mind may we now consider
in detail four of the more acceptable mechanisms which have
been advanced to explain the anti-hypertensive action of the
β-blocking drugs.

(a) Reduction in Cardiac Output (C.O.) The most prominent
effect of β-blockers on the circulation is a lowering of heart
rate and C.O., to an extent that is determined by the patients

level of cardiac sympathetic drive when the compound is first
administered and by the degree of i.s.a. of the drug. The fall
in C.O. appears to be maintained for as long as treatment is
continued. However, although Lydtin et al (29) reported that
the anti-hypertensive action was related to the lowering of C.O.,
other studies (30,31) have failed to confirm this. In fact,
practolol is reported to be almost as effective an anti-
hypertensive as propranolol without producing a concurrent fall
in C.O. (31). It is now generally accepted that simple
reduction in C.O. does not explain the anti-hypertensive action
of the β-blockers (3).

(b) Suppression of Renin Release. Renin is a proteolytic
enzyme mainly secreted by the kidney. It acts on its substrate
(an α-2-glycoprotein, angiotensinogen) to give a decapeptide
angiotensin I which is subsequently degraded to the
physiologically active octapeptide, angiotensin II. Angiotensin
II is a potent vasoconstrictor and, through stimulation of
aldosterone production, leads to retention of Na^+ and water by
the kidney. Thus, both actions of angiotensin II are
hypertensive. Renin release is controlled by renal blood flow
and by the level of Na^+. There is also a fine control exerted
by the sympathetic nervous system which appears to be mediated
via a β-type receptor. For example administration of
isoprenaline produces a rise in renin level which is prevented
by β-blocking agents. The rise in renin following a change in
posture (lying to standing) is also blocked (though not
completely) by β-blockers.

Buhler et al (32) observed that patients with high plasma
renin values generally responded well to propranolol while those
with abnormally low values responded poorly Figure 9. More
recent studies have confirmed that the plasma renin value is
a useful index to those patients who are more likely to respond
to β-blocking therapy. Figure 10 shows the results from a trial
by Amery et al using ICI 66082 (20)

Since it has been reported that hypertensive patients with
high plasma renin levels suffer a higher incidence of vascular
complications, the use of β-blocking drugs would seem to be
particularly beneficial to this class of patient (33).

Although a high level of plasma renin appears to identify
a subject likely to respond to β-blockers the relationship
between the reduction in renin level and fall in blood pressure
is still obscure. While some investigators claim good
correlations between the reduction in renin and blood pressure
others find no such correlation (20). In fact, Stokes et al (34)
showed that pindolol was able to maintain the fall in blood
pressure produced by chronic administration of propranolol
without maintaining the reduction in renin.

A further difficulty to be explained in relating fall in
renin to fall in blood pressure is the timing of the two events.

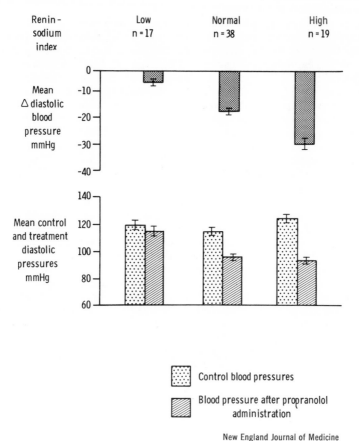

Figure 9. Changes in diastolic blood pressure induced by propranolol in 74 patients (32)

Figure 10. Anti-hypertensive effect
of ICI 66082 (300 mg daily) in hypertensive patients, divided according to
their plasma renin concentration determined recumbent in the morning
(from J. Meekers, A. Missotten, R.
Fagard, D. Demuynck, C. Harvengt,
P. Pas, L. Billiet, and A. Amery in
Archives Internationales de Pharma-
codynamie et de Therapie)

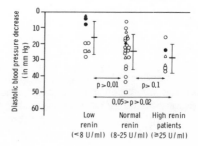

Inhibition of sympathetically mediated increases in renin
immediately follows the administration of a β-blocking drug,
whereas the fall in blood pressure takes some time to occur.

(c) Central Mechanism. Intracerebroventricular (ICV)
administration of propranolol to anaesthetised and to conscious
animals causes an initial transient rise followed by a prolonged
fall in blood pressure. Figure 11 shows this effect for ICV
administration of (-) propranolol to the conscious rabbit. (35)
That the pressor effect is due to the m.s.a. of propranolol and
the depressor to the β-blocking activity is clearly demonstrated
by the administration of (+) propranolol. This isomer shows
m.s.a. but no β-blocking activity and, as is shown in Figure 12.
it produces only a pressor effect (35). Day and Roach compared
the effects of a range of β-blocking drugs following ICV
administration to the conscious cat (36). All the compounds
brought about a fall in blood pressure. The depressor effect
was preceeded by a transient pressor effect with all the
compounds except ICI 66082. It is concluded that the pressor
effect results from m.s.a. or i.s.a. or a combination of the two
since all the drugs except ICI 66082 exhibit one or other, or
both, of these properties.

Table 7. ICV Administration of β-blockers to Conscious
                    Normotensive Cats

Compound	dose (mg)	mean fall b.p. (mm Hg)
propranolol	1.0	30
alprenolol	1.0	26
pindolol	1.0	22
practolol	4.0	20
oxprenolol	0.5	14
sotolol	1.0	22
ICI 66082	2.0	15

(data from Day and Roach 1974)

It is difficult to draw firm conclusions about the
relevance of this central action of β-blockers in animals to
their clinical anti-hypertensive activity bearing in mind that
brain concentrations of the different drugs varies widely

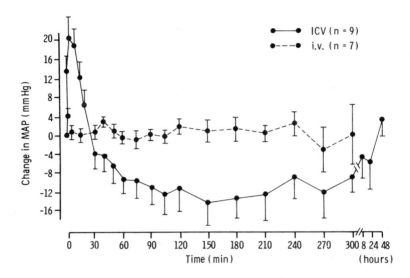

Journal of Pharmacology and Experimental Therapeutics

*Figure 11.   Changes in mean arterial pressure ($\pm$S.E.) in conscious rabbits
after 500 μg of 1-propanolol ICV and i.v. (35)*

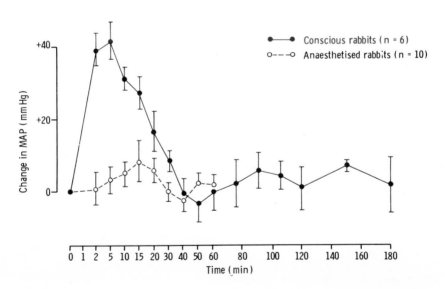

Journal of Pharmacology and Experimental Therapeutics

*Figure 12.   Changes in mean arterial pressure ($\pm$S.E.) after ICV injection of 500
μg of d-propranolol to conscious rabbits and rabbits anaesthetized with sodium
pentobarbital (35)*

following oral (or parenteral) administration. Penetration to
the C.N.S. appears to be related to the lipophilicity of the
molecule. Thus, if a centrally mediated action was an important
component in the anti-hypertensive activity of the β-blockers,
one might expect a compound of low lipophilicity such as
ICI 66082 to be only poorly effective. It is in fact one of the
best.

        Another difficulty is that a centrally mediated action
would not explain the clinically observed time delay to the
onset of the hypotensive effect.

(d) Indirect Lowering of Peripheral Resistance - (20) The
immediate haemodynamic consequences of β-blockade are a fall in
cardiac output accompanied by a rise in total peripheral
resistance (T.P.R.) with the blood pressure remaining virtually
unaffected. This immediate rise in T.P.R. is probably due to a
reflex in α-adrenergic activity in response to the fall in C.O.
If β-blockade is maintained, C.O. remains at the low level, while
in the responsive group, blood pressure falls in association
with a decline in peripheral resistance. These effects are
clearly illustrated by the study carried out by Tarazi and
Dustan (31) and are summarised in Figure 13. More recent
studies would strongly suggest however that the time scale
shown should be shortened to days, or even less. A recent
study with ICI 66082 (20) clearly demonstrates that the full
antihypertensive action is apparent within 48 hours of beginning
treatment Figure 14 (although there is perhaps a suggestion of a
further reduction particularly of diastolic pressure occuring
over the new few days).

        One noteworthy point emerging from this study was that
blood pressure did not return to normal until some two to
three weeks after medication was stopped. This might indicate
that β-blockade has some effect on the hypertensive process
itself.

        It therefore seems likely that the anti-hypertensive action
of the β-blocking drugs is in some way associated with the
decline in peripheral resistance which had initially been
elevated as a response to a reduction in cardiac output. The
precise mechanism responsible for the fall in total peripheral
resistance is as yet unknown. We do know however that the
majority of untreated hypertensives show an excessive sympathetic
response to stimulae such as stress and exercise. It has been
clearly shown that the substantial rise in blood pressure
experienced by hypertensive patients following exercise is
prevented by β-blocking drugs (20). It could be therefore that
it is simply the blockade of surges in cardiac output and blood
pressure which leads to a relaxation of the vascular bed and the

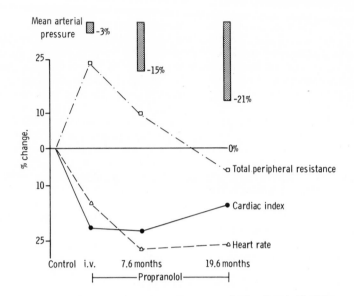

*Figure 13.   Sequential changes with intravenous and long-term
Propranolol therapy in the same 10 hypertensive patients (31)*

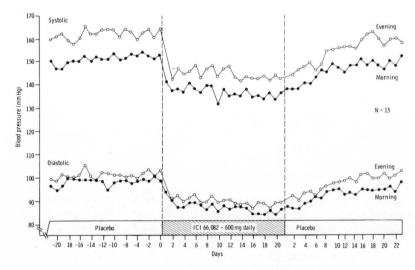

Figure 14.   Effect of ICI 66082 (Tenormin) on blood pressure

subsequent hypotensive effect   (i.e. an action akin to bed rest).
This mechanism of action unlike the previously discussed
ones, would account for the delay in onset of the hypertensive
action. It would also fit in well with the results from the
comparative studies, that provided sufficient drug is given to
adequately block the cardiac β-receptors, all β-blockers are
roughly equally effective. A further point which may possibly
explain why the cardioselective drug ICI 66082 is marginally
more effective than the non-selective propranolol, is that the
former could assist the relaxation of the peripheral vessels
by not blocking the vascular β-receptors.

The relevance of either the experimentally demonstrated
central hypotensive action of the β-blockers, or their ability
to antagonise sympathetically mediated renin release remains
to be proven. While it is still possible that the mechanism
of the anti-hypertensive action of the β-blocking drugs could
contain both a central and a renin-inhibitory component, the
clinical evidence would appear to rule against the possibility
of either being a major component of the mode-of-action.

Thus the "ideal" anti-hypertensive β-blocking agent should
be a moderately long acting cardioselective agent showing little
or no intrinsic sympathomimetic activity.

References

1. Fitzgerald, J.D., Acta Cardiologica, (1972), Suppl. XV, 199.
2. Prichard, B.N.C. and Gillam, P.M.S., Brit. Med. J., (1964),
    2, 725.
3. Conway, J., "Modern Trends in Cardiology 3", Oliver, M.F.,
    ed., Butterworths (London), (1974), p. 376.
4. Ahlquist, R.P., Am. J. Physiol., (1948), 153, 586.
5. Lands, A.M., Arnold, A., McAuliff, J.P., Luduena, F.P. and
    Brown, T.G., Nature (London), (1967), 214, 597.
6. Powell, C.E., and Slater, I.H., J. Pharmac. Exptl. Ther.,
    (1958), 128, 480.
7. Black, J.W., and Stephenson, J.S., Lancet ii, (1962), 311.
8. Barrett, A.M., "Recent Advances in Cardiology", 6th Ed.,
    Hamer, J. ed., Churchill Livingstone (Edinburgh), (1973),
    p. 289.
9. Ariens, E.J., Ann. N.Y. Acad. Sci., (1967), 139, 606.
10. Crowther, A.F., and Smith, L.H., J. Med. Chem., (1968), 11,
    1009.
11. Augstein, J., Cox, D.A., Hane, A.L., Leeming, P.R., and
    Snarey, M., J. Med. Chem., (1973), 16, 1245.
12. Hansch, C., Fujita, T., J. Amer. Chem. Soc., (1964), 86,
    1616.
13. Barrett, A.M., Carter, J., Fitzergerald, J.D., Hull, R.,
    and Le Count, D., Brit. J. Pharmacol., (1973), 48, 340P.
14. Ablad, B., Carlsson, E., and Ek, L., Life Sci. I, (1973),
    12, 107.

15. Richards, W.G., Clarkson, R., and Ganellin, C.R., Proc. Roy. Soc., (in press).
16. Brittain, R.T., Jack, D. and Ritchei, A.C., Advances in Drug Res., (1970), 5, 197.
17. Vaughan-Williams, E.M., Bagwell, E.E., and Singh, B.W., Cardiovasc. Res., (1973), 7, 226.
18. Hellenbrecht, D., Lemmer, B., Weithold, G., and Grobecher, H., Naun, Schmied, Arch. Pharmacol., (1973), 277, 211; Wiethold, G., Hellenbrecht, D., Lemmer, B., and Palm, D., Biochem, Pharmacol., (1973), 22, 1437.
19. Linden, R.J., and Harry, J.D. in "Progress in Cardiology", Eds. Yu, P.N., and Goodwin, J.F., Lea and Febliger, Philadelphia, (1974), p. 227.
20. For a more detailed treatment see Amery, A., and Conway, J., in "Central Actions of Hypotensive Drugs", Dollery, C.T., and Davies, D.S., eds., (1975) Pitman.
21. Bengtsson, C., Acta Med. Scand., (1972), 192, 415.
22. Berglund, G., and Hansson, L., Acta. Med. Scand., (1973), 193, 547.
23. Franciosa, J.A., Conway, J., and Freis, E.D., Circulation, (1973), 48, 118.
24. Lohmoller, G., Frohlich, E.D., Europ. J. Clin. Invest., (1973), 3, 251.
25. Zacharias, F.J., see reference 20.
26. Zacharias, F.J., private communication.
27. Morgan, T.O., Doyle, A.E., Anavekar, S.N., Sabto, J., and Louis, W.J., Postgrad. Med. J., (1974), 50, 253.
28. Kincaid-Smith, P., Am. J. Cardiol., (1973), 32, 575.
29. Lydtin, H., Kusus, T., Daniel, W., Schierl, W., Ackenheil, W., Kempter, M., Lohmoller, H., Niklas, G., And Walter, I., Am. Heart J., (1972), 83, 589.
30. Birkenhager, W.H., Kraus, X.H., Shalekamp, M.A.D.H., Kolsters, G., and Kroon, B.J.M., Folia med. Neerl., (1971), 14, 67-71.
31. Tarazi, R.C., and Dustan, H.P., Am. J. Cardiol., (1972), 29, 633.
32. Buhler, F.R., Laragh, J.H., Vaughan, E.D., Brunner, H.R., Gavras, H., and Baer, L., Am. J. Cardiol., (1973), 32, 511; see also New Engl. J. Med., (1972), 287, 1209.
33. Brunner, H.R., Laragh, J.H., Baer, L., Newton, M.A., Goodwin, F.T., Krakoff, L.R., Bard, R.H., and Buhler, F.R., New Engl. J. Med., (1972), 286, 441.
34. Stokes, G.S., Weber, M.A., and Thornell, J.R., Brit. Med. J. (1974), 1. 60.
35. Reid, J.L., Lewis. P.J., Myers, M.G., and Dollery, C.T., J. Pharm. Explt. Therap., (1974), 188, 394.
36. Day, M.D., and Roach, A.G., Clin. Explt. Pharmacol. Physiol., (1974), 1, 333.

Centrally Acting Antihypertensive Agents

WOLFGANG HOEFKE

Department of Pharmacology, C. H. Boehringer Sohn, Ingelheim, W. Germany

To show how complex it is to influence high blood pressure with therapeutic agents some information on the physiology of blood pressure regulation is given (Fig. 1). The process of regulating blood pressure can be compared with a physical control system where intravascular pressure is the controlled process which has an output variable continuously measured by a feedback transducer - the arterial baroreceptors providing afferent information for the controlling system in the central nervous system - in short "the blood pressure regulating system in the medulla oblongata". In the controlling system a set level of blood pressure serves as a standard for comparison with the measured input of the system, and the difference between the two provides a signal for the autonomic effector, which in turn influences the controlled process.

Besides the arterial baroreceptors, central projections from other inputs, for example cardiac mechano-receptors, chemo-receptors, pulmonary stretch receptors, and somatic inputs, are capable of influencing the controlling system and thereby the autonomic effectors.

There is another system involved in blood pressure regulation: the renin-angiotensin-aldosterone system (Fig. 2). The arterial blood pressure in the kidney influences intrarenal baroreceptors which together with the sodium load at the macula densa lead to renin liberation, angiotensin formation and aldosterone secretion, which by influencing the sodium balance changes the blood volume and influences the arterial blood pressure.

The anatomical structures involved in the maintenance and regulation of the arterial blood pressure are briefly the following (Fig. 3): 1. the arterial wall, 2. the adrenergic receptors, 3. the post-ganglionic

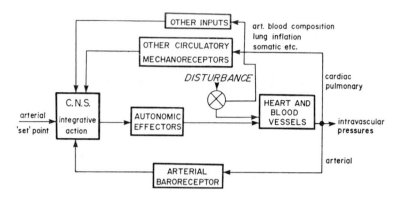

Physiological Reviews
Figure 1.   Circulatory control system (1)

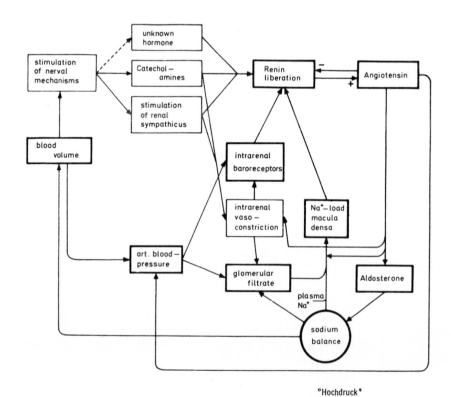

"Hochdruck"
Figure 2.   Renin–angiotensin–aldosterone system (2)

part of the adrenergic neuron and the sympathetic nerve
ending, 4. the sympathetic ganglion and 5. autonomic
structures in the central nervous system. As already
mentioned, all these structures are linked by one or
more controlling systems. By influencing one or the
other part of these systems the regulation may change
in such a way that the blood pressure falls. My lecture
primarily deals with substances influencing these autonomic structures in the CNS.

I should like to talk first about methyldopa (Fig.
4). It is well known that after stimulation of a sympathetic nerve, noradrenaline is liberated at the nerve
ending. These noradrenaline molecules combine with α-
adrenoceptors and are then decomposed by catechol-O-methyl-transferase (COMT) or monoamine-oxydase (MAO) or
for the most part go back into the nerve ending (reuptake) or into the tissues (diffusion) (fig. 5). Phenyl-
alanine and l-tyrosine which circulate in blood are
precursors of the catecholamines. Tyrosine is taken up
into the nerve ending. With the aid of tyrosine hydroxylase, l-dopa is synthesised and dopamine is formed by
decarboxylation through the action of dopa-decarboxylase. Dopamine is then converted to noradrenaline through
the action of dopamine-ß-hydroxylase. The noradrenaline
is stored inside the granules in combination with ATP
(fig. 6). When methyldopa was found clinically to be an
antihypertensive agent as reported by OATES, GILLESPIE,
UDENFRIEND and SJOERDSMA (3), it was thought that the
blood pressure lowering effect of methyldopa was due to
competitive blocking of dopa-decarboxylase and subsequent inhibition of noradrenaline synthesis. Biochemically methyldopa is converted to α-methylnoradrenaline which replaces noradrenaline as a sympathetic transmitter substance. The same holds for α-methyl-meta-tyrosine and α-methyl-para-tyrosine which biochemically are
changed to metaraminol or α-methyl-octopamine. The
blood pressure lowering capacity in man after intravenous treatment with α-methyl-meta-tyrosine has been
shown by HORWITZ and SJOERDSMA (4). With α-methyl-para-
tyrosine clinical results have been disappointing
SJOERDSMA (5)). CARLSSON and LINDQVIST (6) were the
first to indicate that under treatment with methyldopa
α-methylnoradrenaline and not noradrenaline is possibly
released from the storage granules. On the basis of similar findings DAY and RAND (7) were able to present
the theory that stimulation of nerves causes α-methylnoradrenaline to be released from the storage granules
of the sympathetic nerve endings as a false transmitter
substance. This is based on their findings that α-methylnoradrenaline is 2 - 8.5 times less potent than

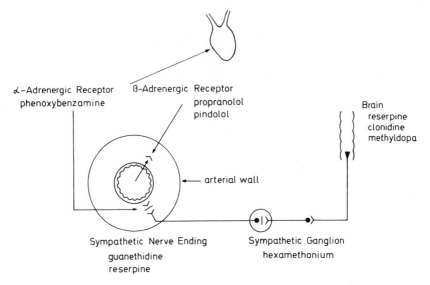

Figure 3.   Anatomical structures involved in circulatory regulation

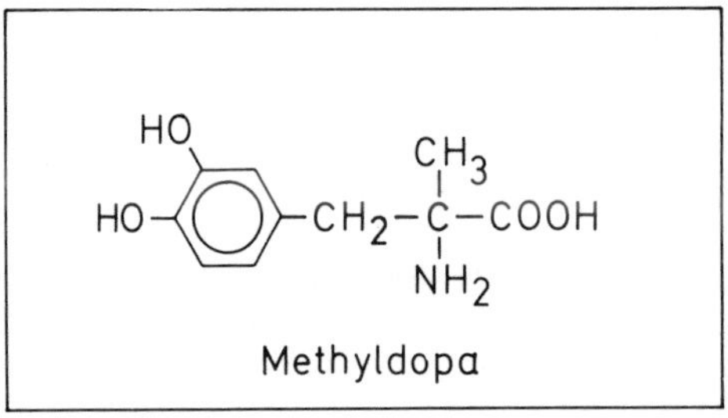

Figure 4.   Chemical structure of methyldopa

Figure 5. Schematic of nerve ending and effector cell. 1, liberation of noradrenaline (NA); 2, reuptake; 3, combining with α-adrenergic receptor; 4, diffusion; 5, degradation of NA. MAO = monoamineoxydase, COMT = catechol-O-methyl-transferase.

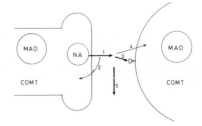

noradrenaline in widely differing test models. The theory of DAY and RAND had been disputed by several workers who have been unable to establish a less potent biological activity of α-methylnoradrenaline, among them PALM et al., (8). Experiments done by HENNING and van ZWIETEN (9) with infusions of methyldopa into a peripheral vein or into the vertebral artery of cats revealed the fact that the lower doses given centrally were more effective than peripheral administration of larger doses. These, as well as experiments done by INGENITO et al. (10), indicate a central mode of action.

At this juncture, a new substance appeared on the scene, namely clonidine (fig. 7), of which I shall now give you a more detailed profile, as I was closely involved in the development of this compound (HOEFKE and KOBINGER (11)). Tests carried out on dogs exhibited a complex influence of clonidine on the circulation as can be seen in fig. 8. A transient rise in blood pressure is followed by a lasting fall. Increasing the dose causes a more distinct rise in blood pressure which might even conceal the hypotensive activity. Hypertensive and hypotensive actions are accompanied by bradycardia. The nictitating membrane is contracted depending on the dose. The carotid sinus reflex produced by clamping both common carotid arteries causes an increase in blood pressure brought about by the decrease in pressure within the region of the carotid sinus. Clonidine has a dose-dependent inhibitory effect on this reflex.

It can now be seen that an immediate peripheral action on the alpha-receptors of the sympathetic nervous system cause vasoconstriction, contraction of the nictitating membrane, increase in the hematocrit, and mydriasis. Clonidine is effective following pretreatment with reserpine which causes discharge of neural noradrenaline and, at the same time, inhibits peripheral effects of the sympathetic nervous system. Moreover, the above-mentioned effects can be blocked by alpha sympatholytic agents such as phentolamine and phenoxy-benzamine. Analysis of the hypotensive as well as bradycardic actions of clonidine exclude to a large extent the possibility of a peripheral vasodilating action, peripheral inhibitory action on the heart and ganglionic blocking activity (HOEFKE and KOBINGER (11), KOBINGER and HOEFKE (12), KOBINGER and WALLAND (13).

The hypotensive action of clonidine could not be explained satisfactorily by effects on the peripheral circulation. Numerous studies therefore considered the possibility of an effect on the central nervous system. Investigations performed on spinalized animals could

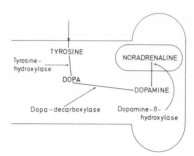

*Figure 6.   Schematic of noradrena-
line synthesis in a sympathetic nerve
ending*

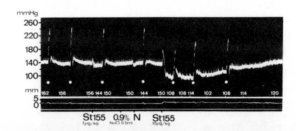

*Figure 7.   Chemical struc-
ture of clonidine*

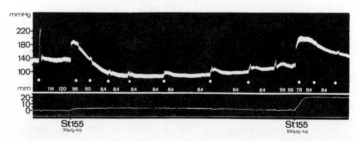

Arzneimittelforschung

*Figure 8.   Cardiovascular effects of clonidine (St 155) in an anaes-
thetized dog. Upper curve, blood pressure, heart frequency. Lower
curve, nictitating membrane. At the whole dots carotid sinus occlusion
reflex was elicited (11).*

provide the answer. The cervical part of the medulla
was cut and thereby the brain function of these animals
was eliminated. If the site of action is located in the
brain, neither a fall in blood pressure nor bradycardia
will occur after spinalization and this is actually
what happened after administration of clonidine (fig.
9). On the contrary, clonidine causes an even more distinct rise in blood pressure in the peripheral circulation after spinalization. Fig. 10 illustrates that
injection of 1 µg/kg clonidine into the cisterna cere-
bellomedullaris of a cat causes a lasting fall in blood
pressure and bradycardia, whereas intravenous injection
of the same dose is distinctly weaker in its effect. It
is assumed that substances injected into the cisterna
reach the fourth ventricle via the foramen Magendi and
Luschka and then pass on to the medulla oblongata. KO-
BINGER (15) is of the opinion therefore that bradycardia as well as decrease in blood pressure and inhibition of pressor circulatory reflexes are caused by an
action on the sympathetic vasomotor center of the medulla oblongata. Investigations carried out by SATTLER
and van ZWIETEN (16) provide further evidence of an
action on the CNS. Low concentrations of clonidine in-
fused into one of the vertebral arteries caused a fall
in blood pressure and bradycardia, whereas hardly any
effect at all could be observed following infusion of
the same doses into one of the peripheral veins.
SCHMITT and coworkers (17) performed tests on dogs re-
cording the electrical activity of sympathetic nerves
before and after administration of clonidine in order
to obtain a more exact analysis of the reduction of
central sympathetic tone. On administration of clonidine a decrease in the frequency of action potentials was
observed in the splanchnic nerve and the cardiac sympathetic nerves. SCHMITT and SCHMITT (18) carried out
further tests in order to localise the hypotensive and
sympathetic inhibitory effects. The experiments in cats
and dogs in which the CNS had been ablated in the area
of the brain stem above the medulla oblongata - have
shown that the clonidine action is maintained. However,
after ablation below the medulla oblongata neither a
decrease in blood pressure nor bradycardia could be
produced by clonidine any longer. According to these
results the medulla oblongata can be regarded as the
main site of action of the hypotensive and bradycardic
effects of clonidine.

Further investigations on the site of action of
clonidine in the spinal cord have been performed by AN-
DÉN and coworkers (19). Injection of dopa caused in
rats an intensified polysynaptic flexor reflex of the

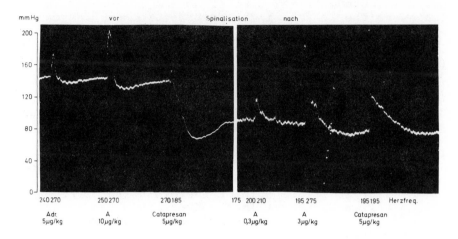

Monatsblätter für Augenheilkunde

Figure 9.   Blood pressure and heart rate under the influence of clonidine before and after spinalization in a cat. Spinalization was done between the two parts of the figure. Adrenaline (Adr.) and clonidine (Clonidin) were given i.v. (14).

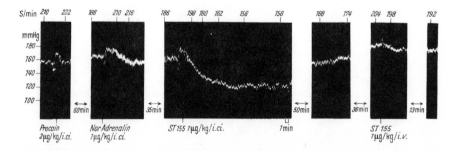

Naunyn–Schmiedeberg's Archives of Pharmacology

Figure 10.   Blood pressure and heart frequency in an anaesthetized cat with sectioned vagi and pretreatment with atropine (1 mg/kg). Decrease of blood pressure and heart rate in beats/min (S/min) after intracisternal (i.ci.) and intravenous (i.v.) injection of clonidine (15).

extremities. Such an effect of dopa can be blocked by alpha-adrenolytic agents, for example phenoxybenzamine. Phenoxybenzamine does not influence the synthesis of noradrenaline from dopa; therefore it must be assumed that phenoxybenzamine blocks adrenergic alpha-receptors in the spinal cord as it does in the periphery of the body. The authors used this model for testing clonidine and found that clonidine similar to dopa causes an intensification of the flexor reflex; this effect can be abolished by alpha-adrenolytic agents. The animals were pre-treated with reserpine in order to exclude the possibility of the effect being brought about by release of noradrenaline. Furthermore, to exclude noradrenaline synthesis by the precursors, appropriate blocking agents were administered.

Further work by SCHMITT and coworkers (20) has supported the hypothesis that adrenergic alpha-receptors do occur inside the CNS and that they are stimulated by clonidine. By intracisternal administration of the alpha-adrenolytic substance piperoxan the authors succeeded in abolishing in cats and dogs the decrease in blood pressure as well as the decrease in heart rate which had been caused by clonidine given intracisternally. Whereas the peripheral alpha-receptors stimulated physiologically by noradrenaline cause vasoconstriction, stimulation of the central alpha-receptors causes a decrease in blood pressure. Noradrenaline cannot penetrate the blood-brain barrier but if it is given intracisternally, an action is exerted on central alpha-receptors, causing a reduction in blood pressure. Piperoxan again produced an antagonistic effect.

Now let us go back to methyldopa. The afore-mentioned experiments by HENNING and van ZWIETEN (21) indicated a central mode of action. HEISE and KRONEBERG (22), perfusing part of the third and the entire fourth ventricle of the brain in cats with methyldopa, α-methyldopamine and α-methylnoradrenaline were able to show a decrease in blood pressure. These effects were significantly blocked by pretreatment with yohimbine and to a lesser extent by phentolamine. These experiments support the concept of blood pressure lowering by an action on central α-adrenoreceptors.

The fact that the modes of action of clonidine and α-methylnoradrenaline are similar to the mode of action of the physiological transmitter noradrenaline indicates the importance of the role of the latter in the central control of blood pressure. It may be mentioned that l-dopa too, the precursor of noradrenaline, penetrates the blood-brain barrier and causes hypotension and bradycardia after systemic administration, when do-

pa-decarboxylase is inhibited extracerebrally by α-hy-
drazino-α-methyl-ß-(3,4-dihydroxyphenyl)-propionic acid
(HENNING and RUBENSON (23)). The same action can be
seen after intraventricular administration of l-dopa
(BAUM and SHROPSHIRE (24). Experiments by HENNING et
al. (25), similar to those of SCHMITT (26) with mid-
collicular transection of the brain in rats showed that
l-dopa - after peripheral dopa-decarboxylase blockade -
reduced blood pressure in the same order as in intact
animals and after spinalization was no longer active.
    In the integration of cardiovascular regulation in
the so-called "medullary vasomotor centre" two different areas for pressor and depressor activity are involved. The main part of the depressor area is the nucleus tractus solitarii, which is rich in noradrenaline
nerve terminals (DAHLSTRÖM and FUXE (27)). Ablation of
this area leads to hypertension in rats (DOBA and REIS
(28)), while stimulation of this area causes hypotension and bradycardia. The same holds true for microin-
jections of noradrenaline into this area (de JONG
(29)). This area is also involved in the carotid sinus
occlusion reflex, which can be blocked by clonidine, as
already mentioned. Recently HAEUSLER (30) has shown
that the action of clonidine bears similarity to a central activation of the depressor baroreceptor reflex
which was elicited by electrical stimulation of the
sinus nerves.
    An essential part of the reduction of the blood
pressure and bradycardia can be explained by central
inhibition of sympathetic tone. However the parasympathetic system is also involved in cardiovascular control. A decrease in blood pressure and bradycardia can
be produced by clonidine even after inactivating the
vagus nerve. SCRIABINE and coworkers (31), however,
have shown that the effect of clonidine in anesthetized
dogs is weaker after inactivation of the vagus nerve.
ROBSON and KAPLAN (32) also came to the conclusion that
clonidine might cause bradycardia by intensification of
vagal reflexes. KOBINGER and WALLAND (33) demonstrated
that clonidine influences vagal reflexes as well. Injection of vasopressor substances such as noradrenaline
and angiotensin cause reflex bradycardia mediated via
the vagus nerve. Such a bradycardia is reinforced if
clonidine is given intracisternally, and the reinforce-
ment can be blocked by phentolamine administered intracisternally.
    Destruction of central adrenergic neurons by in-
traventricular injection of 6-hydroxydopamine (6 OHDA)
virtually abolished the hypotensive effect of methyldopa. Adrenergic neurons are probably required to con-

vert methyldopa to α-methylnoradrenaline which is the
active agent. This is proved by the fact that after
pretreatment with the central dopamine-ß-hydroxylase
inhibitor FLA 63, methyldopa shows no blood pressure
decreasing properties (HAEUSLER and FINCH (34)). In the
case of clonidine, pretreatment with 6 OHDA does not
reduce the blood pressure lowering activity according
to HAEUSLER and FINCH (34) and WARNKE and HOEFKE (35).
This is contrary to the results obtained by DOLLERY and
REID (36). Also after pretreatment with reserpine and
blocking of noradrenaline synthesis with α-methyl-para-
tyrosine clonidine retains its action on the sympathetic system (HAEUSLER (37)). The same holds true for the
intensification of vagally mediated reflex bradycardia
by clonidine (KOBINGER and PICHLER (38)).

Recent experiments carried out by BOLME and coworkers (39) now raise the question of whether the receptors involved in reducing blood pressure are epinephrine receptors or noradrenaline receptors. These workers
found that in rats small doses of yohimbine and piperoxan blocked the blood pressure lowering effect of clonidine, but did not influence the clonidine-induced increase in flexor reflex activity. This effect on the
reflex mechanism is possibly mediated by noradrenaline
receptors which can be blocked only by higher doses of
α-adrenolytic agents. HÖKFELT et al. (40) consider that
epinephrine terminals possibly innervate noradrenaline
cell bodies at the locus coeruleus.

MUJIC and van ROSSUM (41) tested several substituted imidazolines used as nasal decongestants. These
are specific sympathomimetic agents with a direct action on the α-adrenergic receptors. They proved to be
more potent than the naturally-occurring noradrenaline.
Clonidine, which was originally synthesised as a nasal
decongestant, also has strong α-adrenergic activity.
Among the substances which were extensively investigated by van ROSSUM (41) is tetrahydrozoline. HUTCHEON
et al. (42) found that in anaesthetised dogs tetrahydrozoline decreased the blood pressure after an initial
increase and simultaneously caused bradycardia. No fall
in heart rate was observed in spinal cats indicating a
central mechanism of the pharmacological effects.

Besides the similar biological properties of noradrenaline, clonidine and other imadazoline compounds
there are also similarities in the molecular structure
(fig. 11). I have taken noradrenaline as an example of
a substance acting on α-receptors. According to PULMAN
et al. (43), two distances in the molecule are predominant. A distance D from the cationic centre N^+ to the
centre of the aromatic ring equals 5.1 - 5.2 Å and a

distance H from the cationic centre N^+ to the plane of
the aromatic ring equals 1.2 - 1.4 Å. In clonidine the
free rotation of the benzene nucleus around the C-N
single bond means that two conformational isomers may
exist: the planar conformer and the aplanar conformer
with the rings perpendicular to each other. The aplanar
conformer is given preference since the planar conformer is sterically hindered by the two chlorine atoms in
ortho positions. Using the conformations according to
WERMUTH et al. (44), the distances D= (5.0 - 5.1 Å) and
H= (1.28 - 1.36 Å) can be estimated; these compare well
with those of noradrenaline.

The 2,6-diethyl analogue (St 91) is a substance
which is very similar to clonidine in its chemical
structure (fig. 12). This compound tested in spinal
rats is 2.5 times as effective as clonidine in increasing blood pressure, but fails to show a decrease in
blood pressure after intravenous administration to rabbits (HOEFKE, KOBINGER and WALLAND (45)). A reduction
in blood pressure, however, can be achieved by giving
the compound intracisternally in a dose as low as 0.3
μg/kg (fig. 13). The cause for this seems to be the inability of St 91 to penetrate the blood brain barrier.
One physical factor essential for the penetration of
biological membranes is lipophilic character. When this
was tested, the distribution coefficient (P) between
octanol and phosphate buffer at a pH 7.4 was P = 0.06
for St 91 and P = 3.0 for clonidine. Therefore, distribution coefficients play an important part in determi-
ning the spectrum of pharmacological actions of drugs.

The peripheral and central α-adrenergic activities
of a group of di-substituted clonidine analogues with
different distribution coefficients were estimated by
investigating the blood pressure increase in spinal
rats and the bradycardia after parasympathetic blockade. It can be seen in fig. 14 that the most active
agent in spinal rats is St 91, which however showed ab-
solutely no activity on heart rate. From these data relative activities (clonidine = 1) were calculated and
normal logarithms of the product of the α-adrenoceptor
activity (hypertension in spinal rats) times distribution coefficient were plotted along the x-axis. The
normal logarithms of the central cardiodepressor action
(bradycardia in vagotomised rats) were plotted along
the y-axis. With the exception of St 91 which showed no
central action the correlation of these parameters sup-
ports the hypothesis that a connection exists between
α-adrenergic activity, lipoid solubility and central
action (HOEFKE, KOBINGER AND WALLAND (45), fig. 15).
Another physicochemical parameter which was investi-

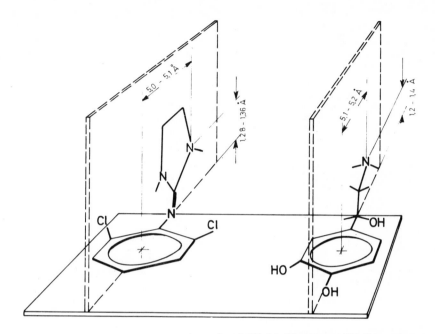

Journal of Medicinal Chemistry and Clinic Therapeutique

Figure 11. Appropriate structures of clonidine and noradrenaline for interaction with the postulated α-adrenergic receptors (on the basis of data from (43) and (44)).

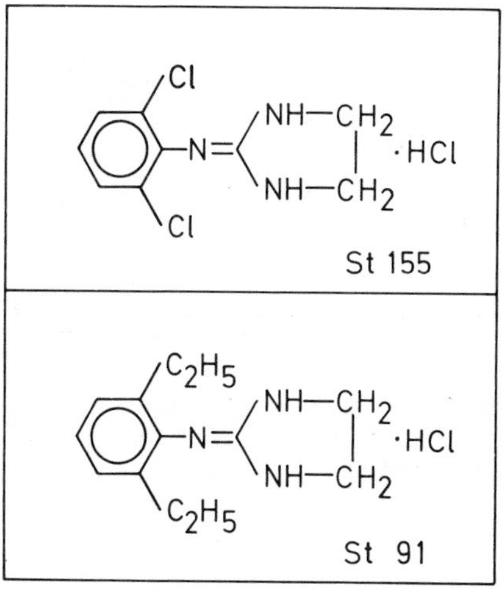

St 155

St 91

Figure 12. Chemical structure of clonidine (St 155) and the 2,6-diethyl-analog (St 91)

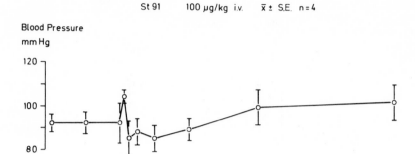

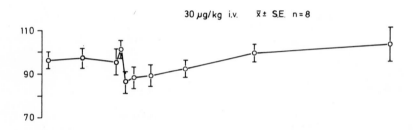

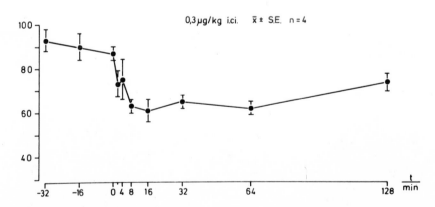

*Figure 13.   Mean blood pressure in anaesthetized rabbits (0.75 g/kg urethan i.p.
and 30 mg Nembutal i.v.) under the influence of St 91 given either intravenously
(i.v.) or intracisternally (i.ci.)*

substance	chemical structure	distribution coefficient octanol / buffer	blood pressure ED$_{30}$ increase in mmHg	heart rate ED$_{50}$ decrease in beats/min
Clonidine (St 155)	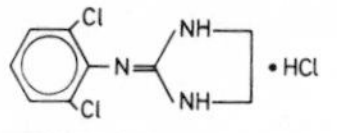 [structure] • HCl	3,0	0,014 mg/kg	0,005 mg/kg
St 91	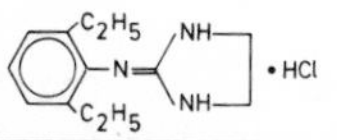 [structure] • HCl	0,06	0,0055 mg/kg	————
St 93	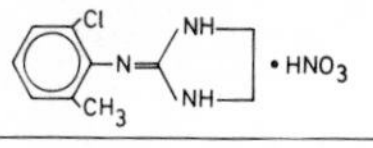 [structure] • HNO$_3$	0,29	0,022 mg/kg	0,0095 mg/kg
Tolonidine (St 375)	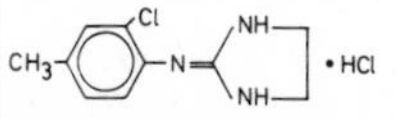 [structure] • HCl	0,11	0,063 mg/kg	0,041 mg/kg
St 600	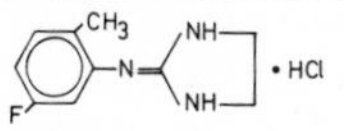 [structure] • HCl	0,15	0,195 mg/kg	0,300 mg/kg
St 608	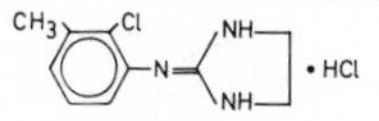 [structure] • HCl	0,27	0,180 mg/kg	0,062 mg/kg

Figure 14. Effects of a group of clonidine derivatives on blood pressure in spinal rats and on heart rate in vagotomized rats. The distribution coefficient was measured with 0.1 m Sörensen phosphate buffer at a pH of 7.4.

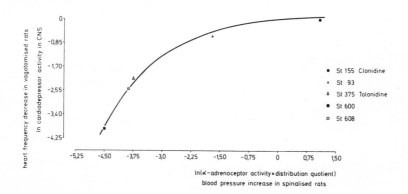

Arzneimittelforschung

Figure 15. Relationship between peripheral α-adrenoceptor activity, lipoid solubility, and centrally mediated cardiodepressor activity. Abscissa: natural logarithms of the product of relative activity on peripheral α-adrenoceptors as derived from blood pressure decreases in spinal rats multiplied by percentage of distribution between octanol/buffer (Figure 4). Ordinate: natural logarithms of the relative CNS activity as derived from bradycardia test in vagotomized rats (45).

gated in connection with the accessibility to central
α-receptors is the pKa. The validity of the correlations between physichochemical parameters and biological activity has, however, yet to be investigated with
other substances. From a more practical point of view
it is possible to test new derivatives of clonidine in
anaesthetised rabbits to ascertain if they have a blood
pressure lowering capacity or not. With this rather
simple method it was possible to evaluate some relationships between chemical structure and pharmacological activity.

The first group of compounds to be investigated
were substituted phenylimino-imidazolines[*]. The introduction of one, two or three chlorine atoms shows maxi-
mal effect with 2,6-dichloro-substitution (fig. 16).
The replacement of chlorine by bromine and trifluoromethyl decreases the hypotensive activity (fig. 17). Al-
ternatively, switching of the two chlorine atoms to
other positions in the phenyl ring also lowers the activity (fig. 18). The same applies to bromine substitution (fig. 19). The substitution with different halogen
or alkyl groups in the 2- and 6-positions leads to a
decrease in the action on blood pressure (fig. 20). The
substitution of alkyl groups in the 2-, 4- and 6-posi-
tions shows no clear cut relationship in structural
activity. While substitution with a methyl and an ethyl
in the ortho-position shows a low activity, the 2-, 6-
di-substituted methyl and ethyl compounds are totally
inactive. The 2-methyl-6-ethyl compound, however is capable of lowering the blood pressure. The 2-, 4-, 6-
trisubstituted derivatives are highly active (fig. 21).
Here again, the distribution coefficient is of importance. The mono-substituted and, to a larger extent di-
substituted compounds show low values for distribution
coefficients between octanol and phosphate buffer at
pH 7.4 whereas the tri-substituted compounds show high
values. Another possibility of variation in the molecule is extension of the bridge between the phenyl ring
and the imidazoline ring. It can be seen in fig. 22
that extension leads to a reduced activity on blood
pressure. The expansion of the imidazoline ring to a
6-, 7- or 8-membered ring as well decreases activity
(fig. 23). Ring closure reactions of 2-imino-imidazoli-
nes lead to annellated bi- and tri-cyclic hetero rings.
Here again the blood pressure lowering activity is re-

---

[*] All the compounds tested were synthesised by Dr. H.
STÄHLE, Dept. of Pharmaceutical Chemistry, C.H.
Boehringer Sohn, Ingelheim, W.-Germany (see also STÄHLE
(46) and POOK et al. (59)).

CHEMICAL STRUCTURE	blood pressure decrease mmHg ED_{20} mg/kg
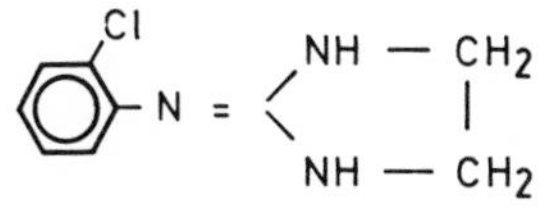	1.00
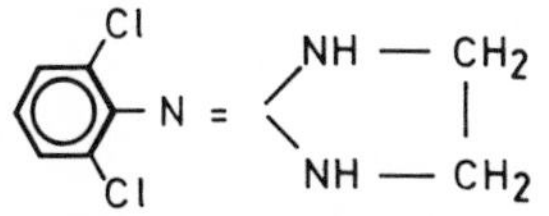	0.01
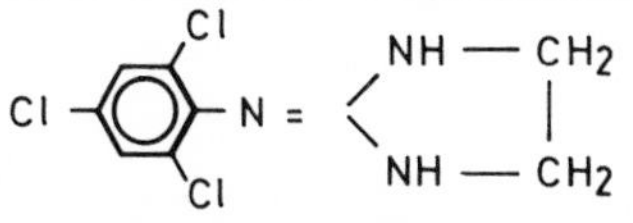	0.09

Figure 16. Influence of one, two, or three chlorine atoms in the phenyl ring on blood pressure in anaesthetized rabbits

CHEMICAL STRUCTURE	blood pressure decrease mmHg ED_{20} mg/kg
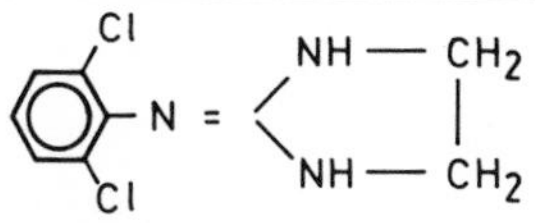	0.010
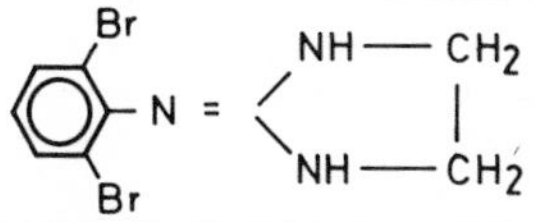	0.045
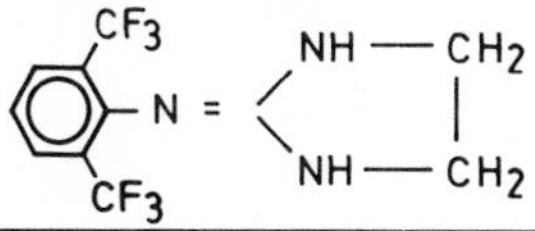	0.060

Figure 17. Effect of replacement of chlorine in 2,6-position of the phenyl ring by bromine and trifluoromethyl on blood pressure

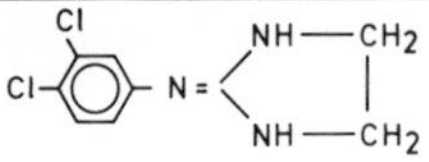

Figure 18. Significance of the position of two chlorine atoms in the phenyl ring on the blood pressure lowering effect

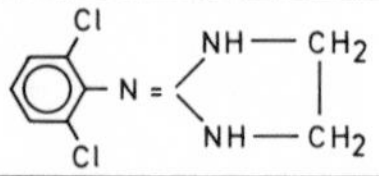

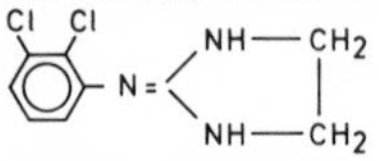

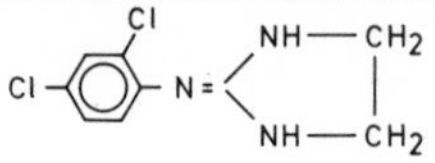

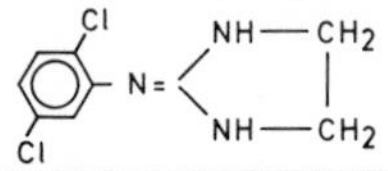

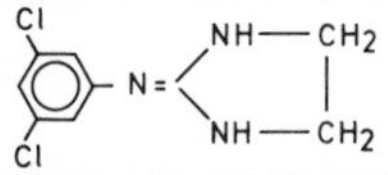

Figure 19. Position of two bromine atoms in the phenyl ring shows similarities in its effect on blood pressure to chlorine substituted phenyl–imino–imidazolines

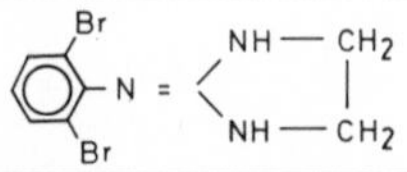

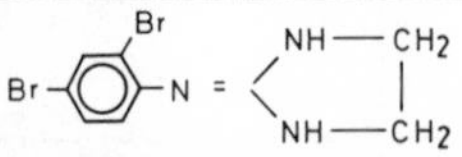

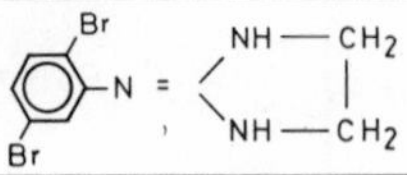

CHEMICAL STRUCTURE	blood pressure decrease mmHg ED_{20} mg/kg
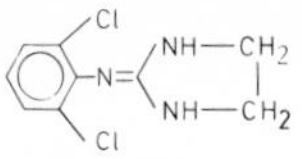 (structure: dichlorophenyl imino-imidazoline, Cl and Cl)	0,01
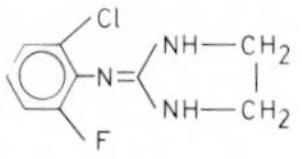 (structure: chloro-fluoro-phenyl imino-imidazoline, Cl and F)	0,04
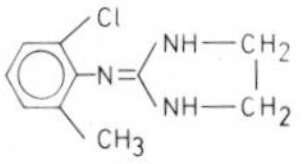 (structure: chloro-methyl-phenyl imino-imidazoline, Cl and CH_3)	0,05
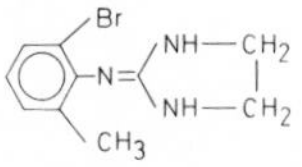 (structure: bromo-methyl-phenyl imino-imidazoline, Br and CH_3)	0,6

Figure 20. Influence of substitution with different halogens and halogen with methyl in the phenyl ring on blood pressure activity

CHEMICAL STRUCTURE	blood pressure decrease mmHg ED_{20} mg/kg
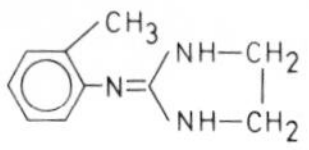 (structure: CH_3 phenyl imino-imidazoline)	1,2
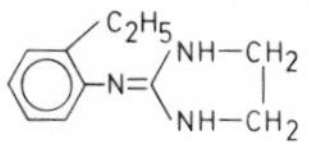 (structure: C_2H_5 phenyl imino-imidazoline)	0,4
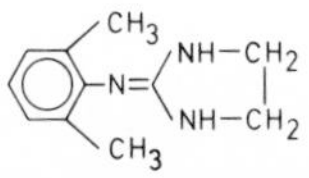 (structure: CH_3, CH_3 phenyl imino-imidazoline)	0
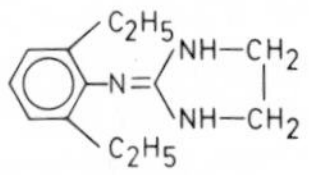 (structure: C_2H_5, C_2H_5 phenyl imino-imidazoline)	0
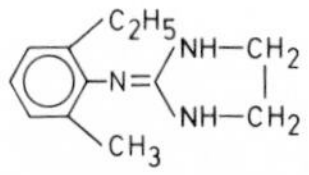 (structure: C_2H_5, CH_3 phenyl imino-imidazoline)	0,3
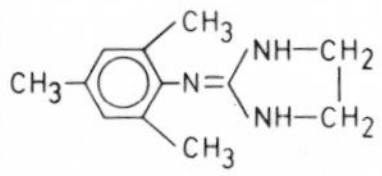 (structure: CH_3-, CH_3, CH_3 phenyl imino-imidazoline)	0,03
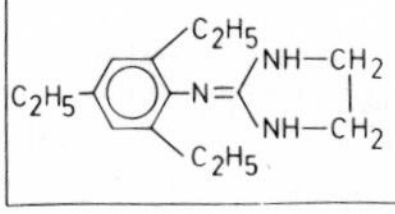 (structure: C_2H_5-, C_2H_5, C_2H_5 phenyl imino-imidazoline)	0,03

Figure 21. Substitution of alkyl groups in the phenyl ring in imino–imidazolines and effect on blood pressure

CHEMICAL STRUCTURE	blood pressure decrease mmHg ED_{20} mg/kg
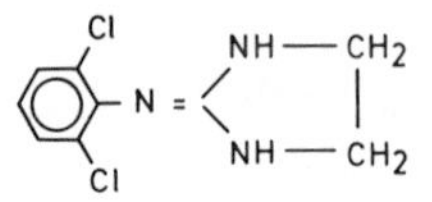	0,0 1
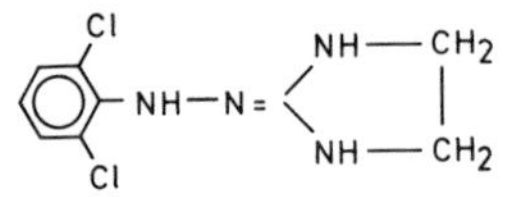	0,2 4
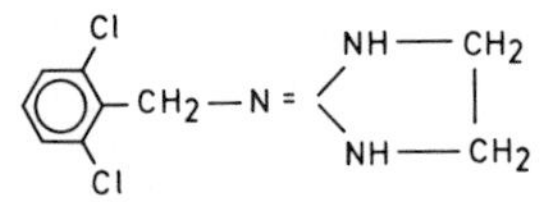	0,8 5
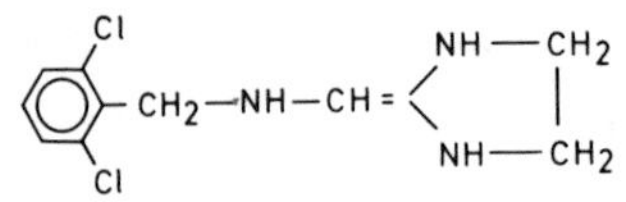	1,0 0

Figure 22. Influence of "bridge extension" between the phenyl and the imidazoline ring on blood pressure lowering activity

CHEMICAL STRUCTURE	blood pressure decrease mmHg ED_{20} mg/kg
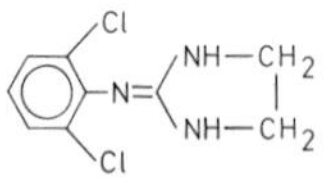	0,01
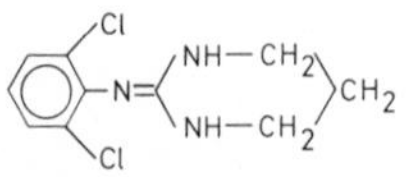	3,0
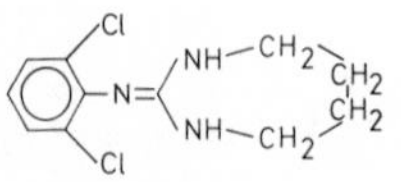	3,0
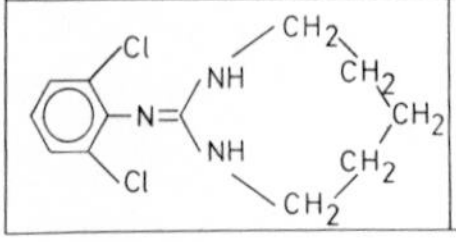	1,0

Figure 23. Effect of extension of the imidazoline ring to six-, seven-, and eight-membered rings on hypotensive activity in rabbits

duced (fig. 24).

In the last few years many substances related to clonidine have been synthesised and tested pharmacologically and clinically all over the world. Examples of these substances can be seen in figs. 25 and 26.

The sedative action of noradrenaline has been known since 1954, when FELDBERG and SHERWOOD (47) injected the substance into the lateral ventricle of cats, thus avoiding the blood-brain barrier. Similar results have been obtained with adrenaline, which LEIMDÖRFER (48) proved to be active in producing deep sleep in man by injecting 2 mg intracisternally. The sedative action of methyldopa is well known from its clinical use.

The sedative effects of clonidine were observed in the very first animal experiments performed (HOEFKE and KOBINGER (11)). Obvious symptoms of sedation can be observed on administration of therapeutic doses to dogs, cats, rabbits, rats and mice. Investigations on the mechanism of the sedative action have mainly been performed on chicks. In chicks only a couple of days old the blood-brain barrier is not yet fully developed. This means that even substances administered to the periphery of the body display an effect on the CNS which can no longer be observed later on. Clonidine induces sleep in these animals, as described by ZAIMIS (49), FÜGNER and HOEFKE (50) and by DELBARRE and SCHMITT (51). Noradrenaline, as well as α-methylnoradrenaline, which cannot permeate the blood-brain barrier in older animals, cause sleep. This effect could be inhibited with phentolamine in the case of noradrenaline and also in the case of clonidine (FÜGNER (52)). Therefore it may be assumed, that here again central adrenergic alpha-receptors are involved.

Another clinically important effect I would like to mention is the inhibition of salivary secretion by clonidine. Both the sympathetic nervous system and the parasympathetic nervous system are involved in the physiological regulation of salivation. HOEFKE (53) as well as RAND and coworkers (54) found that parasympathetic salivary secretion stimulated by electrical impulses on the chorda tympani and by carbachol could not be blocked by clonidine in anaesthetised animals. In our own experiments in rats with clonidine and the 2,6-diethyl derivative St 91 which does not penetrate to the CNS, secretion of saliva was blocked only after clonidine, (HOEFKE (55)) indicating a central mode of action.

When looking for new compounds it is important to show if there is any differentiation between the reduc-

CHEMICAL STRUCTURE	blood pressure decrease mmHg ED_{20} mg/kg
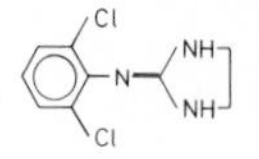	0,01
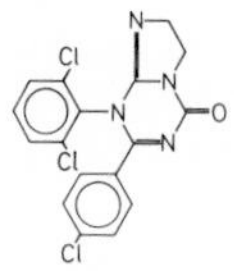	0,2
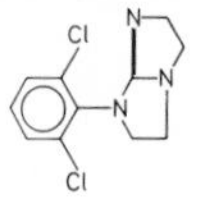	0,3
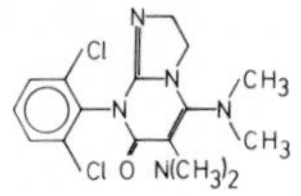	1,5

Figure 24. Hypotensive activity of clonidine derivatives with annelated hetero-rings

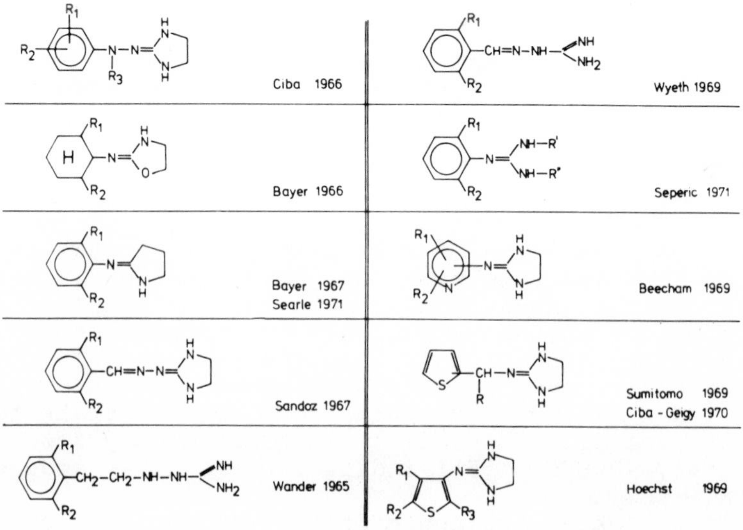

Medicinal Chemistry IV

Figure 25. Survey of compounds structurally related to clonidine (46)

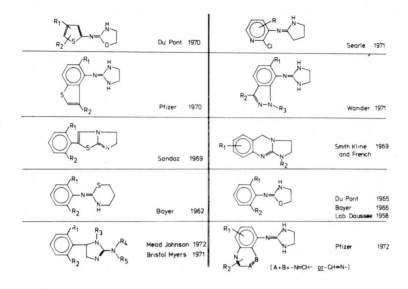

Medicinal Chemistry IV

Figure 26.   Survey of compounds structurally related to clonidine (46)

	antihypertensive and sympathomimetic action			central sedation		gastric secretion	
	antihypertensive a. rat ED_{20}mg/kg	sympatho-mimet. a. rat ED_{50}mg/kg	quotient s/a	sleep effect chick ED_{50}mg/kg	quotient c/a	Shay rat ED_{50}mg/kg	quotient g/a
Cloni-dine	0,04	0,009	0,23	0,06	1,5	0,04	1,0
St 600	0,5	0,039	0,078	1,95	3,8	7,5	15,0
St 608	0,8	0,3	0,38	0,81	1,0	4,0	5,0

Life Sciences

Figure 27.   Comparison of the relationship between antihypertensive and sympathomimetic activity and sedation and inhibition of gastric secretion of clonidine and two derivatives (St 600 and St 608). The antihypertensive activity was tested in genetic hypertensive rats. The sympathomimetic activity was measured as blood pressure increase in spinal rats. The sleep effect in chicks was tested according to the method in Reference 50, and the gastric secretion in rats was measured according to the method in Reference 57.

CHEMICAL STRUCTURE	dose mg/kg i. p.	decrease in blood pressure mmHg
HO—⬡—CH$_2$—C(CH$_3$)(NH$_2$)—COOH	2 0 0	- 7 0
HO—⬡(CH$_3$)—CH$_2$—C(CH$_3$)(NH$_2$)—COOH	3 0 0	0
HO—⬡(CH$_3$)—CH$_2$—C(CH$_3$)(NH$_2$)—COOH	3 0 0	0
HO(CH$_3$)—⬡—CH$_2$—C(CH$_3$)(NH$_2$)—COOH	2 0 0	0
H$_3$CO—⬡—CH$_2$—C(CH$_3$)(NH$_2$)—COOH	3 0 0	0
HO—⬡—CH$_2$—C(CH$_3$)(NH—CH$_3$)—COOH	3 0 0	0

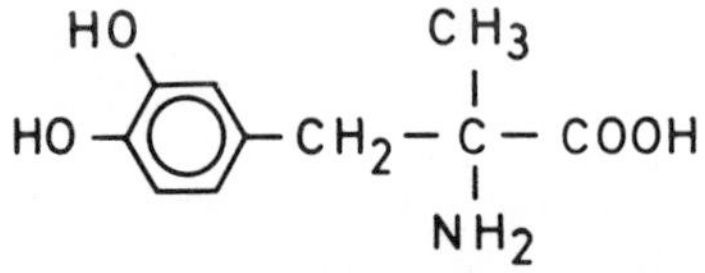

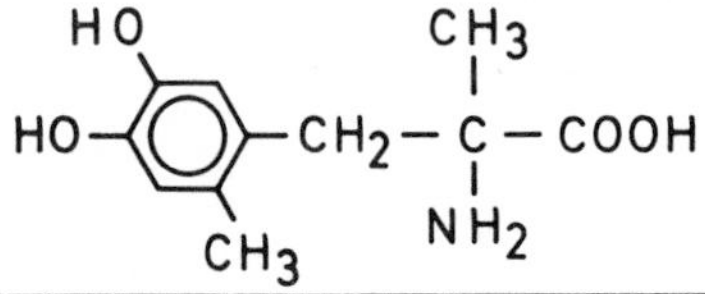

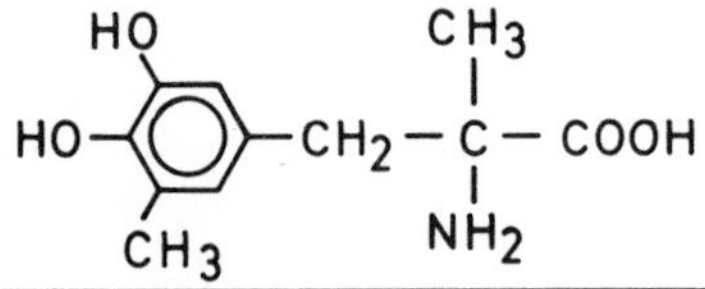

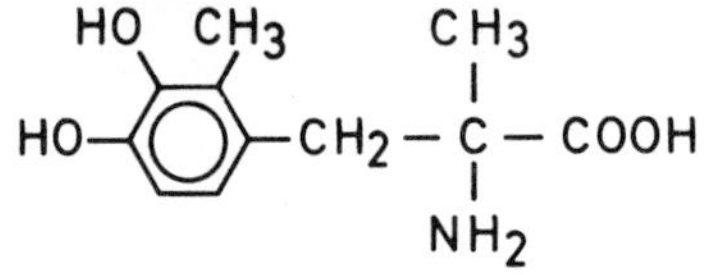

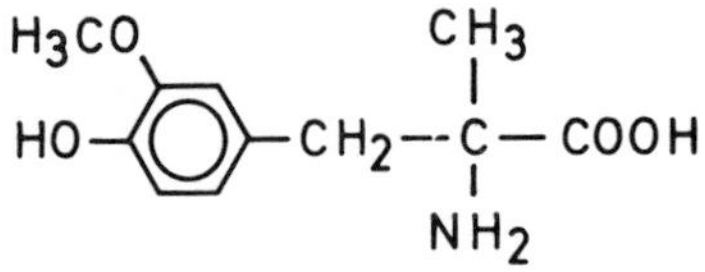

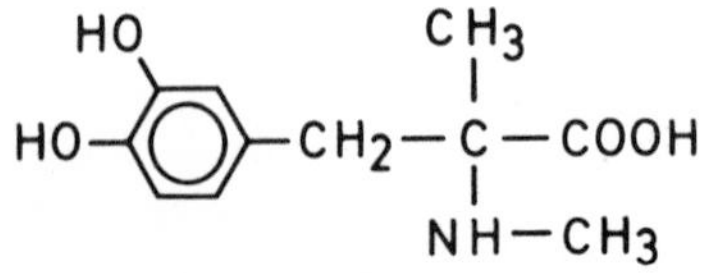

Figure 28. *Influence of an additional methyl group in derivatives of methyldopa on the blood pressure lowering activity in spontaneously hypertensive rats*

tion in blood pressure and the sedation and the inhibition of secretion. For screening purposes it is easier to test the effect on secretion in rats according to the method of SHAY et al. (56), because in rats gastric secretion is largely dependent on the volume of saliva (LEVINE (57), STOCKHAUS and WICK (58)). It can be seen in fig. 27 that secretion and sedation are both influenced less by St 600 than by clonidine; with St 608 only the effect on salivary secretion was reduced.

The effect on the blood pressure by these compounds can be explained by an action on central α-receptors. But from the aforementioned facts it can be assumed that the sedation and reduction in salivation are dependent also on an influence on central α-receptors.

Now to return to methyldopa. It has to be converted to α-methylnoradrenaline before it is effective. α-methylnoradrenaline, however, unlike methyldopa, is not able to penetrate the blood-brain barrier.

It is more difficult to look for active substances here because the precursor must be able to penetrate the blood-brain barrier. α-amino-acids must be decarboxylated, and the amines must be active on an order similar to noradrenaline. Further the substance should show no activity outside the CNS. For years substances were synthesized and tested under the auspices of the "false transmitter theory", but no one was able to prove its efficacy in clinical practice. One example from our own experiments is given in fig. 28. The introduction of one additional methyl-group either on the phenyl ring or replacing one hydrogen of the hydroxyl group or on the amino group, did not produce substances which are able to lower the blood pressure when high doses were tested in genetically hypertensive rats.

It is to be hoped that scientific results will soon give us new leads to even more effective antihypertensive agents.

Literature Cited
1. KORNER, P.J.: Physiological Reviews 1971, 51, 312
2. BOCK, K.D.: "Hochdruck" Thieme, Stuttgart 1969
3. OATES, J.A., L. GILLESPIE Jr. S. UDENFRIEND and A. SJOERDSMA: Science 1960, 131, 1890
4. HORWITZ, D. and A. SJOERDSMA: Life Sci. 1964, 3, 41
5. SJOERDSMA, A.: Circulation Res. 1967, 21 Suppl. III., 119
6. CARLSSON, A. and M. LINDQVIST: Acta physiol. scand. 1962, 54, 87
7. DAY, M.D. and M.J. RAND: J. Pharm. Pharmacol. 1963, 15, 224
8. PALM, D., W. LANGENECKERT and P. HOLTZ: Naunyn-

Schmiedebergs Arch. Pharmakol. exp. Path. 1967, 258, 128

9. HENNING, M. and P.A. van ZWIETEN: J. Pharm. Pharmacol. 1967, 19, 403
10. INGENITO, A.J., J.P. BARRETT and L. PROCITA: J. Pharmacol. Exper. Therap. 1970, 175, 593
11. HOEFKE, W. and W. KOBINGER: Arzneimittelforschung 1966, 16, 1038
12. KOBINGER, W. and W. HOEFKE: in "Hochdrucktherapie" ed. HEILMEYER, L., H.J. HOLTMEIER and E.F. PFEIFFER, 4 Thieme, Stuttgart 1968
13. KOBINGER, W. and A. WALLAND: Arzneimittelforschung 1967, 17, 292
14. HOEFKE, W.: in "Clonidin in der Augenheilkunde" Bücherei des Augenarztes, Beiheft der klin. Monatsblätter für Augenheilkunde 1974, 63, 4
15. KOBINGER, W.: Naunyn-Schmiedebergs Arch. Pharmak. exp. Path. 1967, 258, 48
16. SATTLER, R.W. and P.A. van ZWIETEN: Europ. J. Pharmacol. 1967, 2, 9
17. SCHMITT, H., H. SCHMITT, J.R. BOISSIER and J.F. GIUDICELLI: Europ. J. Pharmacol. 1967, 2, 147
18. SCHMITT H. and H. SCHMITT: Europ. J. Pharmacol. 1969, 6, 8
19. ANDÉN, N.E., M. CORRODI, K. FUXE, B. HÖKFELT, T. HÖKFELT, C. RYDIN and F. SVENSSON: Life Sci. 1970, 9, 513
20. SCHMITT, H., H. SCHMITT and S. FENARD: Europ. J. Pharmacol. 1971, 14, 98
21. HENNING, M. and P.A. van ZWIETEN: J. Pharm. Pharmacol. 1968, 20, 409
22. HEISE, A. and G. KRONEBERG: Naunyn-Schmiedebergs Arch. Pharmacol. 1972, 279, 452
23. HENNING, M. and A. RUBENSON: J. Pharm. Pharmacol. 1970, 22, 553
24. BAUM, T. and A.T. SHROPSHIRE: Neuropharmacol. 1973, 12, 49
25. HENNING, M., A. RUBENSON and G. TROLIN: J. Pharm. Pharmacol. 1972, 24, 447
26. SCHMITT, H.: in "Catapres in Hypertension" Ed. CONOLLY, M.E. 23 Butterworth, London, 1970
27. DAHLSTRÖM, A. and K. FUXE: Acta physiol. scand. 1964, 62, Supp. 232
28. DOBA, N. and D.J. REIS: Circulation Res. 1973, 32, 584
29. DE JONG, W.: Europ. J. Pharmacol. 1974, 29, 179
30. HAEUSLER, G.: Naunyn-Schmiedebergs Arch. Pharmacol. 1974, 282, R 29
31. SCRIABINE, A., C.A. STONE and J.M. STARVORSKI: Pharmacologist 1968, 10, 156

32. ROBSON, R.D. and H.R. KAPLAN: Europ. J. Pharmacol. 1969, 5, 328
33. KOBINGER W. and A. WALLAND: Europ. J. Pharmacol. 1971, 19, 210
34. HAEUSLER, G. and L. FINCH: J. Pharmacol. (Paris) 1972, 3, 544
35. WARNKE, E. and W. HOEFKE: In preparation
36. DOLLERY, C.T. and J.L. REID: Brit. J. Pharmacol. 1973, 47, 206
37. HAEUSLER, G.: Naunyn-Schmiedebergs Arch. Pharmacol. 1974, 286, 97
38. KOBINGER, W. and L. PICHLER: Europ. J. Pharmacol. 1974, 27, 151
39. BOLME, P., H. CORRODI, K. FUXE, T. HÖKFELT, P. LID-BRINK and M. GOLDSTEIN: Europ. J. Pharmacol. 1974, 28, 89
40. HÖKFELT, T., K. FUXE, M. GOLDSTEIN and O. JOHANNS-SON: Brain Research 1974, 66, 235
41. MUJIC, M. and J.M. van ROSSUM: Arch. int. Pharmaco-dyn. 1965, 155, 432
42. HUTCHEON, D.E., A. SCRIABINE and V.N. NIESSLER: J. Pharmacol. Exper. Therap. 1958, 122, 101
43. PULMAN, B., J.L. COUBEILS, Ph. COURRIÈRE and J.P. GERVOIS: J. Med. Chem. 1972, 15, 17
44. WERMUTH, W.G., J. SCHWARTZ, G. LECLERC, J.P. GARNIER and B. ROUOT: Clinic Therapeutique 1973, 1, 115
45. HOEFKE, W., W. KOBINGER and A. WALLAND: Arzneimit-telforschung 1975, 25, 786
46. STÄHLE, H.: in Medicinal Chemistry IV, Ed. MAAS, J. Elsevier, 75 Amsterdam 1974
47. FELDBERG, W. and S.L. SHERWOOD: J. Physiol. 1954, 123, 148
48. LEIMDÖRFER, A.: Wien. klin. Wschr. 1948, 60, 382
49. ZAIMIS, E.: in Catapres in Hypertension Ed. CONOLLY, E.M. 9 Butterworth, London 1970
50. FÜGNER, A. and W. HOEFKE: Arzneimittelforschung 1971, 21, 1243
51. DELBARRE, B. and H. SCHMITT: Europ. J. Pharmacol. 1971, 13, 356
52. FÜGNER, A.: Arzneimittelforschung 1971, 21, 1350
53. HOEFKE, W.: unpublished data 1967
54. RAND, M.J., M. RUSH and J. WILSON: Europ. J. Phar-macol. 1969, 5, 168
55. HOEFKE, W.: VI. International Congress of Pharma-col. 1975, Abstracts 119
56. SHAY, H., D.C. SUN and M.A. GRUENSTEIN: Gastro-enterology 1954, 26, 906
57. LEVINE, R.J.: Life Sci. 1965, 4, 959
58. STOCKHAUS, K. and H. WICK: Arzneimittelforschung

1970, 20, 858
59. POOK, K.H., H. STÄHLE and M. DANIEL: Chem. Ber.
    1974, 107, 2644

Antihypertensives Acting by a Peripheral Mechanism

JOHN E. FRANCIS

Research Department, Pharmaceuticals Division, CIBA-GEIGY Corp., Ardsley, N. Y. 10502

The efforts of medicinal researchers in trying to find anti-hypertensive agents working by a peripheral mechanism arise from the expectation that these agents will effect good blood pressure control without the central nervous system side effects which are observed to some extent with every marketed agent to date which has a strong central component in its mechanism of action. Since antihypertensive therapy, except in emergency treatment, requires drug treatment every day for a long period of time, perhaps decades, it is important that the mental and physical capabilities of the patient be impaired as little as possible. This is particularly important in those cases where the hypertensive patient feels well despite his condition.

Peripheral Vasodilating Antihypertensive Agents

Peripherally acting drugs have not cornered the major share of the antihypertensive market because of their own set of serious side effects. Agents which act through relaxation of the vasculature, commonly called peripheral vasodilators (even though some peripheral vasodilators do not lower blood pressure), can cause edema and increased sodium and renin levels in the blood as well as reflex tachycardia. Edema and elevated sodium levels can be controlled by co-administration of a diuretic. The more recent finding that the other two side effects can be overcome by β-adrenergic blocking agents has greatly increased the market potential for vasodilating antihypertensives used in combination with diuretics and β-blockers.

Presently on the U.S. market there are three compounds commonly considered as peripheral dilating hypotensive agents. These are hydralazine (I), placed on the market in 1953 by CIBA, diazoxide (II) from Schering in 1973 and sodium nitroprusside (III) made available by Roche in 1974.

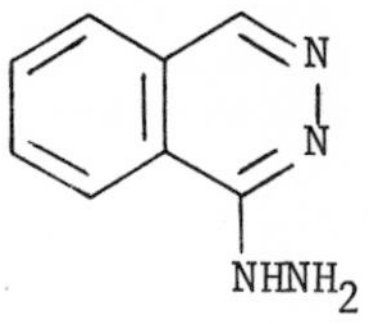

I   II   III

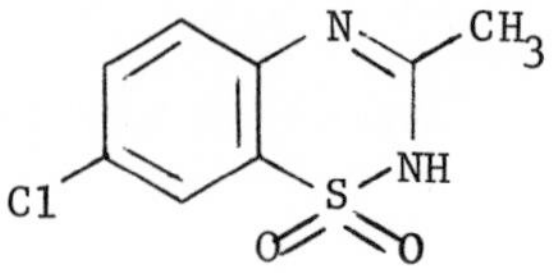

Diazoxide and sodium nitroprusside, relative newcomers to the market, are indicated only for hypertensive emergencies. This leaves hydralazine as the only drug of this kind available to date on the U.S. market for chronic use. The total picture of the mechanism of action of hydralazine is still not clearly defined but there is general agreement that direct relaxation of the vasculature leading to reduced peripheral resistance is the principal component of its mechanism of action. This drug has stood the test of time despite such side effects as headache, tachycardia and a syndrome which resembles acute systemic lupus erythematosus, often called "hydralazine syndrome" (1).

Many attempts have been made to improve hydralazine through structure modification. The early work of the inventor, Jean Druey, at CIBA in Basle, covered many variations of the structure and the structure-activity relationships established by Druey and his co-workers hold to this day (2, 3). The most important compounds were those with the phthalazine (IV) and the pyridazine (V) ring systems.

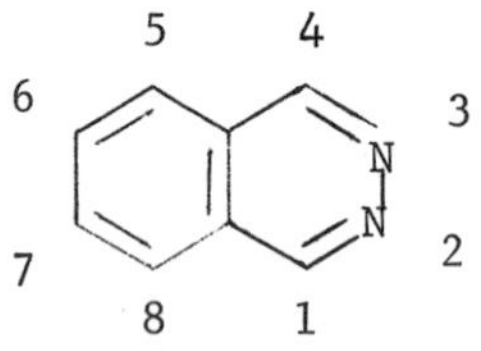

IV 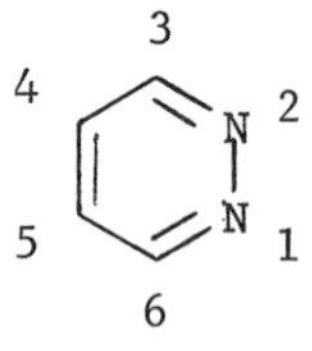   V

The following structure-activity relationships were defined: a) For prolonged hypotensive activity, the hydrazino group must be present in the 1-position of phthalazine or the 3-position of pyridazine. The hydrazino group is the most important structural feature.
b) Activity is retained in many examples where the other carbon atoms are additionally substituted.
c) The benzene ring of phthalazine may be replaced by pyridine.

d) Hydrazones of hydralazine retain activity. Reaction with acids, esters or acid chlorides converts hydralazine to an s-triazolo (3,4-a) phthalazine which is inactive presumably because the hydrazino group is tied up in a stable ring system.

An empirical rule defining the minimum requirements for activity in this type of compound is illustrated by structure VI which shows that the -C=N-N=C- moiety must be in a six membered heteroaromatic system with the hydrazino group (or its hydrazone) attached to one of the carbons.

VI

There are some exceptions to the rule, namely structures VII through XI. All of these were active in animal tests but only 1-hydrazinoisoquinoline (VII) showed activity in man comparable to hydralazine.

VII   VIII   IX

X   XI

Dihydralazine (XII), marketed by CIBA in Europe, shows less acute toxicity in animals than hydralazine (4,5). Ecarazine (XIII), sold by Polfa-Pabiance as Binazin®, is a hydrazide of hydralazine, which may indicate that other acylated derivatives

XII   XIII

may be active also, provided cyclization can be avoided. Pico-dralazine (XIV), a constituent of Vallene Complex®, is sold by Farmasimes in Spain and Hydracarbazine (XV), a constituent of Normatensyl®, is marketed by Theraplix in France.

XIV   X V

New compounds continue to appear in the literature and some are reported to show advantages over hydralazine in animal studies. For example, L-6150 (XVI) is said to be less toxic acutely (6). ISF-2123 (XVII) is more potent in rats and dogs (7). DJ-1461 (XVIII), a hydrazone of hydralazine, is claimed to cause considerably less tachycardia (8). To date it has not been shown that any of these compounds has a significant clinical advantage over hydralazine and therefore, over the last twenty-five years, slight modifications of the hydralazine structure have not produced a better drug of this type.

XVI   XVII   XVIII

Diazoxide (II) has been known since the early 1960's (9) and must be considered as a well known lead. It bears a structural resemblance to the diuretic agent, chlorothiazide (XIX) but, unlike chlorothiazide, it is non-diuretic. Analogs have been prepared by scientists at Schering (10) and by a group in Italy (11). The Italian group reported that compound XX lowers blood pressure and heart rate intravenously in rats but causes

XIX   XX

XXI

atrioventricular block (12). The Schering group has designed pazoxide (XXI), which is more potent than diazoxide in the DOCA rat model. It is interesting that pazoxide was one of the most potent compounds predicted by a multiple regression analysis of a series of 2H-1,2,4-benzothiadiazine-1,1-dioxides (13). Comparison of "calculated" with observed activities in the DOCA rat lead to the conclusion that maximum activity would be expected for compounds with a) highly lipophilic groups at positions 6 and 7, b) a pKa value greater than eight and c) a narrowly defined π factor which is a measure of the effect of the substituent at position 3 and can be calculated from the octanol-water partition coefficient.

Replacement of the $-SO_2-$ moiety of the diazoxide ring system by carbonyl leads to an interesting series of compounds, namely the 4-quinazolinones (XXIIa). Extensive synthetic efforts at Pfizer led to the 2-dialkylamino-6,7-dimethoxy-4-quinazolinones which were particularly promising in dog studies (14). The best of these, compound XXIII, showed good oral activity with no influence on heart rate and no sign of tolerance development. Examination of more than fifty analogs revealed that the 2-aminoid group might be varied to some extent but the

XXIIa   XXIIb   XXIII

6,7-dimethoxy substitution was essential for high activity. Replacement of the methoxyls with alkyl, hydrogen, hydroxyl or even 6,7-methylenedioxy diminishes or eliminates activity. Since substitution at the 3-position eliminates activity, this suggests that the 4-hydroxy-quinazoline structure (XXIIb) may be the active species. Structures XXIV and XXV bridge the gap between

XXIV   XXV

the diazoxide series and the 4-hydroxyquinazoline group but none of these compounds showed activity in the dog at the doses tested (15). Compound XXIII was shown to be active in man but

was subsequently displaced by compounds in the 4-aminoquinazoline
series which were clearly more potent in animal studies (16).
The compounds XXVI through XXIX were reported to be more potent
than hydralazine in dogs.

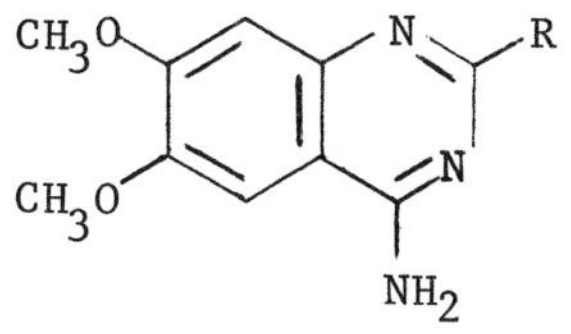

XXVI   R= NMe$_2$

XXVII   R= -N⟩⟨NCH$_2$CH=CH$_2$

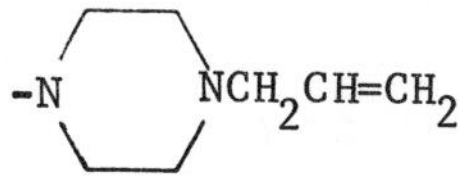

XXVIII R= -N⟩⟨NCOCH$_2$CH⟨CH$_3$ CH$_3$ (O)

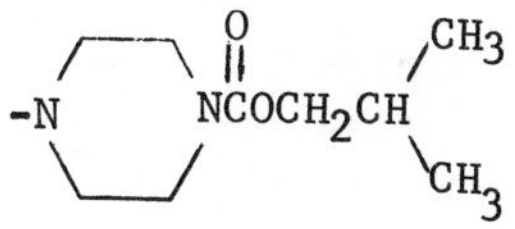

XXIX   R= -N⟩⟨NC- (O, furan)

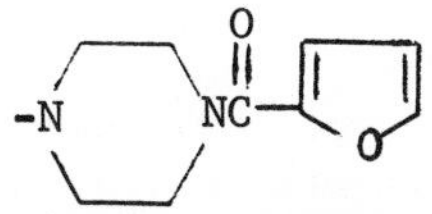

all lowered blood pressure and peripheral resistance without
tachycardia. The piperazines XXVIII and XXIX were the most
potent (20-150 ug/kg orally). Of these four, prazosin (XXIX)
has emerged as a potent antihypertensive agent in clinical trials
(17) and has now been marketed in several countries including
the United Kingdom. Trimazosin (XXX), with three methoxyl
groups in the benzene ring, has also been shown to be clinically
effective, although it appears to be less potent than
prazosin (18).

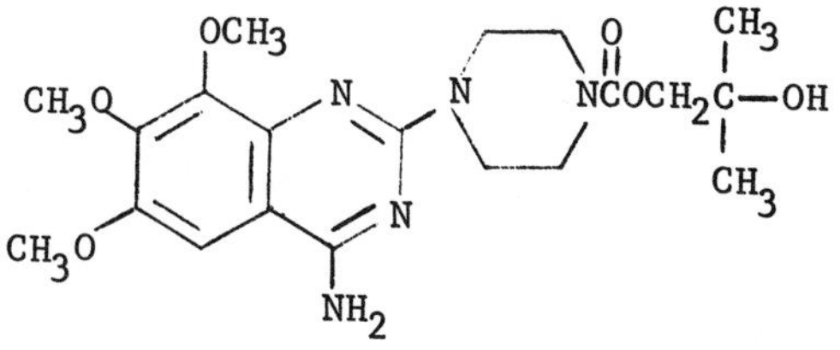

XXX

Another potent peripheral vasodilator with hypotensive
activity is minoxidil (U-10,858, XXXI). The drug was developed
at the Upjohn Corporation, apparently as a follow-up of a
previous clinical candidate, diallylmelamine -N-oxide (U-20,388,
XXXII). The amine precursor, diallylmelamine (U-7720, XXXIII),
is active in rats and dogs but not in man because the active

metabolite is the N-oxide, which does not form in the human
body (19, 20).

XXXI   XXXII   XXXIII

    Clinical reports on minoxidil indicate that the drug is
effective, particularly in cases which are refractory to other
drugs (21, 22). It has the typical side-effects of a vasodilator and co-administration of a diuretic and a β-adrenergic
blocker is recommended in many of the reported studies (21-28).
An unusual and troublesome side-effect, particularly in women,
is lanugal hair growth (21, 22).
    An enzyme inhibitor of microbial origin with a simple
structure, fusaric acid (XXXIV), is a hypotensive agent. This
compound has been tested clinically as the free acid (29) and
as the calcium salt (30) and is orally effective in man with a
low incidence of side-effects. Dopamine-β-hydroxylase inhibitory
action of this compound has been demonstrated in man (29).

XXXIV   XXXV   XXXVI

    Introduction of chlorine or bromine into the 3- and/or
4- positions of the side chain yields more potent compounds in
terms of hypotension in rats and dopamine β- hydroxylase inhibition (31, 32). The analog YP-279 (XXXV) is also hypotensive
in rats but is said not to affect brain norepinephrine biosynthesis unlike fusaric acid or dibromofusaric acid (33-35).
Fusaric acid amide (bupicomide, Sch 10595, XXXVI) is clinically
effective at 300 to 1800 mg per day and is said to have hemodynamic effects similar to hydralazine (36, 37). The amide is

metabolized to the acid in man (38).

Turning from pyridine to dihydropyridine, we find another
interesting structural type represented by SKF 24260 (XXXVII).
In dogs, this compound is a potent, long acting hypotensive
which shows reflex tachycardia but no tolerance potential (39).
It is closely related to the Bayer compound nifedipine currently
under investigation in Europe as an antianginal agent (40).
Both drugs are said to lower blood pressure in man.

XXXVII   XXXVIII

An investigation of more than ninety analogs of XXXVII led
to the following generalizations regarding structure-activity
relationships (41):

a) In general, the best compounds have a cyclic substituent
at the 4-position, particularly ortho-substituted aryl or a
heterocycle.

b) Methyl groups at positions 2 and 6 are preferable to
ethyl or hydrogen.

c) Replacement of the ester groups at positions 3 and 5 by
other electron-withdrawing groups lowers activity.

d) The ethyl esters usually have greater oral potency than
the methyl esters.

e) Substitution at the nitrogen atom lowers activity in
general.

Since the pyridine derivatives obtained as metabolic
products of SKF 24260 are inactive (42), the importance of the
dihydropyridine structure is clear.

A mesoionic compound PR-G-138-Cl (XXXIX) from Pharma
Research in Canada is reported to lower blood pressure in man at
low doses by a vasodilator type mechanism (43). This structure
is related to SIN-10 (XL) which was reported earlier by Japanese
scientists as active in dogs (44). Compounds related to
structure XXXIX were compared in spontaneous hypertensive rats
and those with the oxadiazole ring hydrogen replaced by chlorine
or bromine were as active as the parent compound, although replacement by methyl caused a loss of activity (45).

XXXIX   XL

Drugs Affecting Noradrenergic Mechanisms

Since the discovery that norepinephrine release at the
adrenergic nerve terminal is the mechanism whereby the human
body maintains sympathetic tone, medicinal scientists have
searched for agents which reduce sympathetic tone through interference with norepinephrine peripherally. Reduction of the
effect of norepinephrine should lead to a lowering of blood
pressure which might be achieved in the following ways:
a) Adrenergic blockade: Substances which combine with the
effector cells and make them unresponsive to norepinephrine
cause adrenergic blockade and compounds which appear to inhibit
selectively either α- or β-adrenergic receptors can be identi-
fied.
b) Adrenergic neuronal blockade: In contrast to adrenergic
blockers, these agents act within the sympathetic nerves to
prevent the release of transmitter amine, thus reducing stimulation at the effector cells without decreasing their responsive-
ness.
c) Inhibition of reuptake and storage: Norepinephrine is present
in adrenergic nerve terminals in a bound form in storage vesicles
in equilibrium with an intracellular pool of the free catecholamine. Activation of the neuron liberates norepinephrine into
the synaptic cleft where some of the molecules activate the
receptors but most are rapidly drawn back into the nerve terminal
as the neuron firing ceases. An agent may interfere with the
reuptake of norepinephrine into the nerve terminal thus prolong-
ing the time norepinephrine is present in the synaptic cleft.
The catecholamine may then be inactivated through methylation of
the meta-hydroxyl group catalyzed by the enzyme catechol-0-
methyltransferase. Also, an agent may interfere with reuptake
of norepinephrine into storage vesicles which allows the free
intracellular pool to be depleted by oxidation catalyzed by
monamine oxidase, an enzyme present in mitochondria within the
nerve terminal.

d) Inhibition of biosynthesis: The conversion of tyrosine to norepinephrine via dihydroxyphenylalanine (DOPA) and dihydroxyphenethylamine (dopamine) involves three enzymatically controlled steps. Drugs which inhibit these enzymes could be expected to decrease norepinephrine concentration. Since the first step is rate-limiting, tyrosine hydroxylase inhibition should be the most desirable mechanism.

e) Norepinephrine release: Agents which release norepinephrine from storage sites may cause a short acting sympathomimetic effect, but the long range effect is one of depletion if norepinephrine is metabolized rapidly and not replaced by biosynthesis quickly enough.

f) Displacement of norepinephrine at storage sites: Some amines related in structure to norepinephrine may displace molecule for molecule the natural transmitter in the storage sites. If these amines are less sympathomimetic they should, when released, produce an attenuated effect on adrenergic receptors, resulting in lowering of blood pressure.

Although β-adrenergic blocking agents have only recently been exploited as potential antihypertensive agents, α-adrenergic blockers have been known since the late 1930's and have received early consideration as hypotensive agents. The drugs phentolamine (XLI), piperoxan (XLII) and phenoxybenzamine (XLIII) are three which were studied clinically in depth. These strong α-blocking agents have side effects resulting from the α-blockade,

XLI

XLII

XLIII

namely increased cardiac rate and force, and postural hypotension, and they are not used alone in the treatment of hypertension. Phentolamine and phenoxybenzamine are on the U.S. market for use in the management of pheochromocytoma (46). A successful clinical trial of a combination of phentolamine with the β-adrenergic blocking agent oxprenolol (47), leads to the conclusion that a combination of α- and β-blockers could be a useful method for

controlling blood pressure and thus the α-blocking properties of
a compound need not be feared. Prazosin (vide supra) has an
α-blocking effect, for example (48). Another compound thought
to have a strong α-blocking component as well as a vasodilating
effect is indoramin (XLIV). This indole derivative differs
from other α-blockers in that it depresses cardiac output with
the result that, clinically, tachycardia is not a serious side
effect (49, 50).

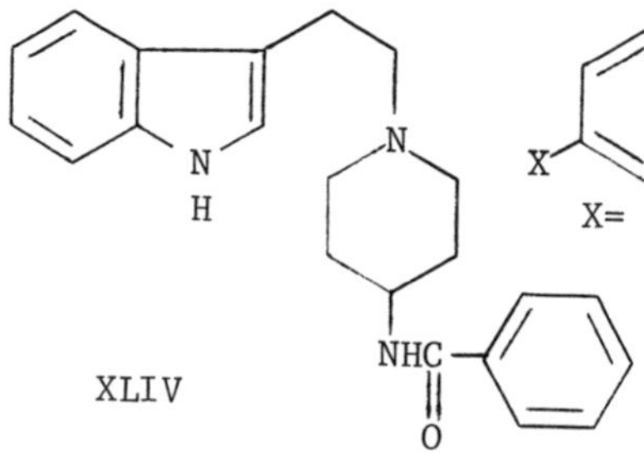

XLIV

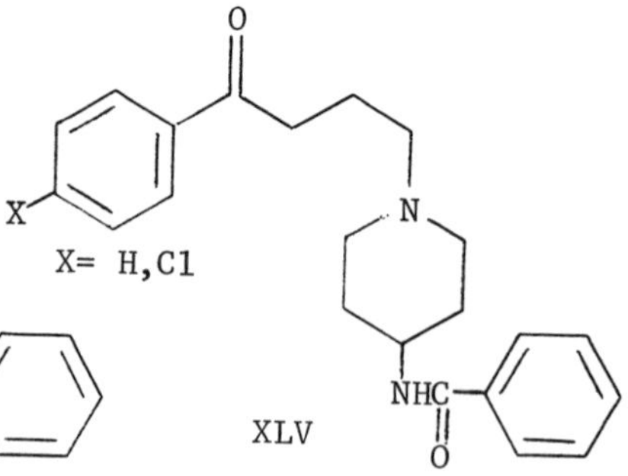

X= H,Cl

XLV

   Indoramin was the product of investigation at Wyeth Laboratories of a number of compounds containing the indolylethyl-
piperidine group. Structure-activity relationships have been
published in detail (51-53). The most remarkable findings appear
to be that no advantage was gained by extensive modification of
the 4-benzamidopiperidine moiety nor by replacement of the indole
group by other heterocycles. Replacement of indolylethyl by
benzoylpropyl (structure XLV: R=H) produced a compound equipotent
in rats and the p-chloro analog was the most potent α-blocker in
the series. The central nervous system side effects of indoramin
may limit its utility and the close resemblance of XLV to known
central nervous system drugs such as haloperidol suggests that
this new series will also have central effects. Nonetheless,
indoramin appears to be an interesting lead and a focal point of
further research.
   Since ergot alkaloids were the first adrenergic blocking
agents to be discovered, it is noteworthy that the ergot derivative nicergoline (XLVI) was marketed in Italy by Farmitalia in
1974, for parenteral treatment of hypertension as well as peripheral and cerebral vasodilatation. It is said to have
α-blocking (54) and vasodilating properties and is well tolerated
with no undesirable side effects on the heart.

XLVI

The Allen and Hanburys compound ibidomide (AH 5158, XLVII) is a combination α- and β-blocker (55, 56). Early clinical trials indicate that it lowers blood pressure in man (57) and although the β-blockade is non-cardioselective, the broncho-constrictor effects appear to be suppressed by the α-blocking component (58). This profile differs markedly from that of the

XLVII   XLVIII

close structural analog nylidrin (XLVIII) which is a β-stimulant possibly effective in vasospastic disorders (59).

The late 1950's and early 1960's saw the emergence of adrenergic neuron blocking agents. Xylocholine (XLIX), structurally similar to the general ganglionic blocking agents, showed some promise as a selective blocker of the peripheral sympathetic system, but since it showed serious cholinergic side effects it was undesirable for use in man (60).

XLIX   L

Bretylium (L) showed selective adrenergic blocking activity in animals and man but erratic absorption and other side effects limited its utility in hypertension (61).

A significant advance in this area was the discovery of the CIBA compound SU-4029 (LI).

LI   LII

This amidoxime reduced blood pressure in renal and neurogenic hypertensive dogs with a slow onset of activity and prolonged action (62). In the clinic, it was hypotensive in man but caused elevation of body temperature (63). Extensive structure modifications by Dr. Robert Mull and co-workers at CIBA in terms of ring size, chain length and end group led to guanethidine (LII) (64). This guanidine had the optimal activity in the series and is much superior in adrenergic neuronal blocking properties to SU 4029. The drug showed a prolonged blood pressure lowering effect in man, even in severe cases, with no tachycardia, as expected for such an agent. This was marketed in 1960 and is still the only drug of its kind on the U.S. market. Further studies in animals showed that norepinephrine depletion occurs in heart but not in brain and consequently central side effects are minimal. Although there is no tachycardia, orthostatic hypotension is a frequent side effect and diarrhea and inhibition of ejaculation are common reactions. The desirable blood pressure lowering effect coupled with these side effects made attempts to improve on guanethidine worthwhile. There have been many hundreds of publications on guanethidine and a vast number of synthetic variations on the structure. By 1967, five compounds related in structure to guanethidine had reached the market in at least one European country (65), namely, guanochlor (Pfizer, LIII), guanacline (Bayer, LIV), guanoxan (Pfizer, LV) bethanidine (Burroughs-Wellcome, LVI) and debrisoquine (Hoffmann-LaRoche, LVII). All of these differ pharmacologically from guanethidine to some extent and each is claimed to show some advantage over guanethidine in man, such as greater activity in patients refractory to guanethidine or better control of blood pressure through more frequent dosage.

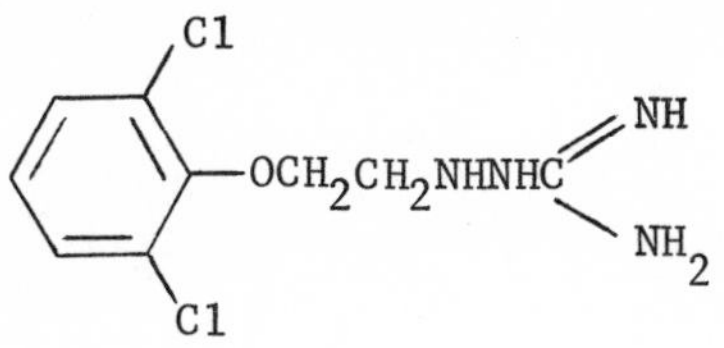

LIII

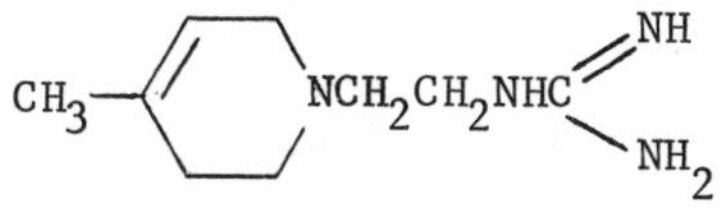

LIV

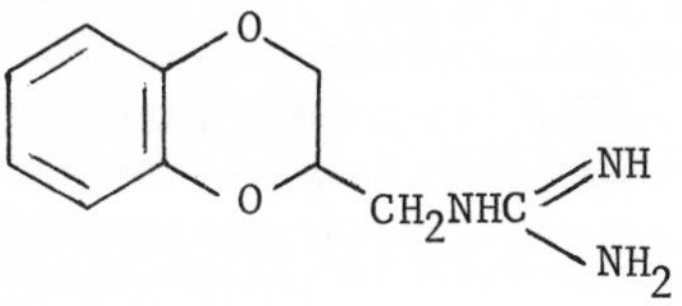

LV

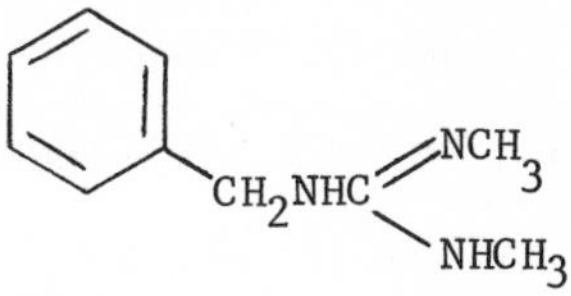

LVI

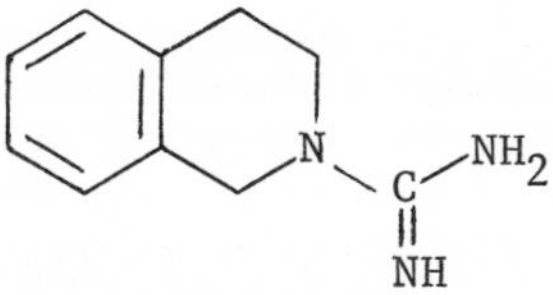

LVII

Inability to gain acceptance on the U.S. market has not dis-
couraged all efforts in this field and three other clinically
effective drugs have been studied extensively, namely guanadrel
(Upjohn, LVIII), guanabenz (Wyeth, LIX) and guancydine (Lederle,
LX).

LVIII   LIX   LX

        Guanadrel is similar to guanethidine but is believed to
cause fewer incidents of diarrhea (66). Guanabenz, a structural
hybrid of guanethidine and clonidine, has a profile of activity
which also appears to be hybrid (67, 68). It lowers blood
pressure without orthostatic hypotension and diarrhea, but it
causes drowsiness, indicative of a central mode of action (69).
At the opposite pole of activity profile is guancydine which
appears to have no significant neuronal blocking activity but
rather a direct vascular effect (70, 71). Lederle scientists
have reported that only the branched chain cyanoguanidines are
significantly active; the guanethidine analog is inactive (72).
The history of the variation of the guanethidine structure
illustrates that molecular modification can bring about vast
changes in mechanism of action while the desired end result
(in this case, hypotension) is still achieved.
        The Rauwolfia alkaloid reserpine, due to its strong central
component of activity, is excluded from this review, even though
it has the peripheral effect of releasing norepinephrine from
storage sites where it can be metabolized by monoamine oxidase.
This results in neurotransmitter depletion and it appears that
good blood pressure control would be achieved by a drug which
has this peripheral mechanism but lacks the central component.
The Mead-Johnson compound MJ-10459-2 (LXI) shows activity in

LXI

several animal models apparently by peripheral norepinephrine
depletion with no effect on brain amines. No clinical reports
have yet appeared but the pharmacological profile in some ways
resembles guanethidine and in others, a "peripherally acting
reserpine" (73-76).

Inhibition of norepinephrine biosynthesis can be achieved
quite well by chronic oral administration of the tyrosine hydroxylase inhibitor α-methyl-p-tyrosine (LXII) but reduction in
blood pressure was not achieved in patients with essential
hypertension (77). Another potent inhibitor, 3-iodotyrosine
(LXIII) was also inactive in man (78). Apparently, substantial
reduction of norepinephrine (50-70%) is not enough to achieve
the desired effect.

When norepinephrine is substituted in the storage sites
by amines of similar structure which are less agonistic, these
agents are called "false transmitters." Until its central

LXII   LXIII

mechanism was defined,   methyldopa (LXIV) was thought by some
to be converted enzymatically to α-methylnorepinephrine (LXV)
which was taken up in peripheral storage sites and subsequently
released to cause blood pressure lowering effects (79, 80) by
the false transmitter mechanism. Two genuine examples of

LXIV   LXV

peripherally acting false transmitters are metaraminol (LXVI)
and p-hydroxynorephedrine (PHN, LXVII), since neither of them
penetrate the blood-brain barrier at effective doses, unlike
the metaraminol precursor, α-methyl-m-tyrosine (LXVIII) (<u>81</u>, <u>82</u>).
Crout and co-workers observed that metaraminol lowered blood

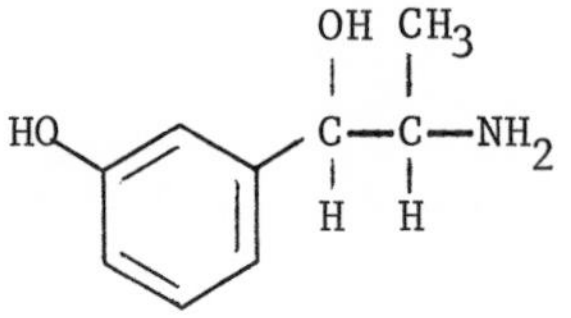

LXVI 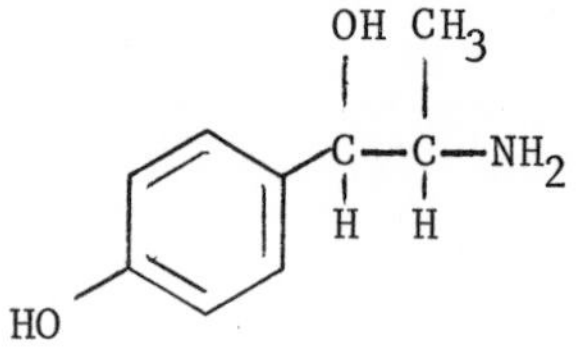   LXVII

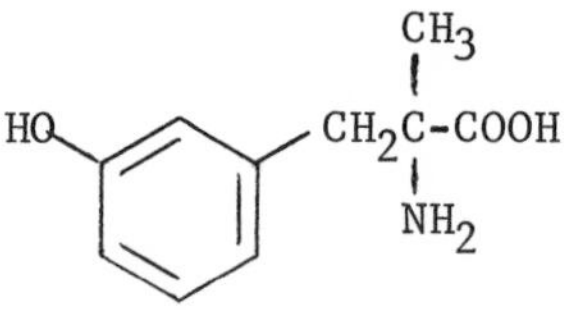

LXVIII

pressure in humans at very low doses (<u>83</u>) without central side
effects, but since slightly higher doses produced strong pressor
effects, the drug could not be used safely. PHN, tested by Oates
and co-workers (<u>84</u>), has the same type of activity but much
weaker potency. This drug also was administered cautiously. To
avoid the inherent pressor activity of metaraminol, scientists
at Merck, Sharp and Dohme prepared a number of ethers of
metaraminol which showed no pressor activity in animals (<u>85</u>).
These ethers were slowly metabolized to metaraminol <u>in vivo</u> and
the false transmitter gradually displaced norepinephrine from
peripheral sites, whereupon blood pressure lowering was achieved.
Like metaraminol, the ethers did not penetrate the brain
appreciably (<u>86</u>). The m-chlorobenzyl ether (LXIX) was the most
promising member of the series studied.

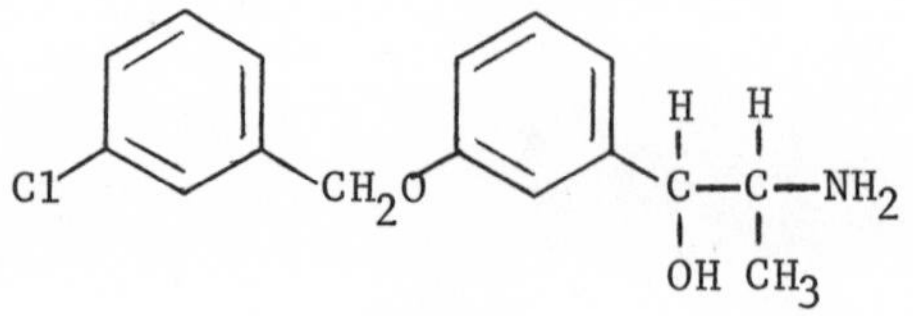

LXIX

Substances Interfering with Angiotensin II

The natural blood globulin, angiotensinogen, is converted by the proteolytic kidney enzyme, renin, to the decapeptide angiotensin I. This substance is not a pressor agent but is cleaved by plasma converting enzyme to the powerful vaso-constrictor angiotensin II, an octapeptide.

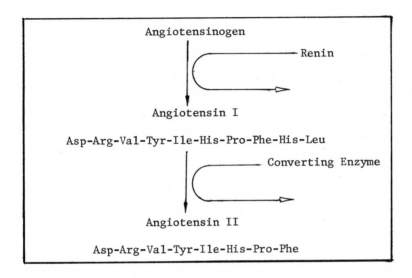

Angiotensin II is believed to trigger a series of events important in blood pressure regulation. Inhibition of the effect of this agent, either through competitive inhibition or interference with its biosynthesis could reveal the role of this peptide and perhaps lead to a different type of antihypertensive therapy. A rational approach to the target of a competitive inhibitor would require the synthesis of a number of peptides differing slightly from the angiotensin II structure followed by biological evaluation. When the Merrifield method of peptide synthesis was developed (87), this approach became a realistic one. Several groups of investigators have prepared competitive inhibitors which look promising in vitro and in animal tests (88-96) but the inhibitor which has attracted the most attention to date is Sar[1]-Ala[8]-angiotensin II, (saralasin, LXX) prepared at Norwich Pharmacal Company (97). When administered by intra-venous infusion in patients with high renin hypertension, the synthetic peptide lowered blood pressure effectively (98).

```
┌─────────────────────────────────────────┐
│                                           │
│              Saralasin                    │
│                                           │
│   Sar-Arg-Val-Tyr-Ile-His-Pro-Ala         │
│                                           │
└─────────────────────────────────────────┘
```

LXX

From an entirely different source, namely, the venom of
the snake <u>Bothrops jararaca</u>, scientists at Squibb isolated a
nonapeptide (SQ 20,881, LXXI) which is a potent inhibitor of
the converting enzyme (<u>99</u>).


```
┌─────────────────────────────────────────────┐
│                                               │
│                 SQ 20,881                     │
│                                               │
│   p-Glu-Trp-Pro-Arg-Pro-Gln-Ile-Pro-Pro       │
│                                               │
└─────────────────────────────────────────────┘
```

LXXI

Comparison of SQ 20,881 with fifty-seven related synthetic
peptides indicated that the last five amino acids of the
sequence are required for significant enzyme inhibiting activity
(<u>100</u>). This nonapeptide, intravenously, lowered blood pressure
even in patients with normal renin levels (<u>101</u>, <u>102</u>). This
effect is strongly augmented by sodium depletion.
  The interest in these peptides and others whose mechanisms
of action are not yet so clearly defined is evident from the
many recent publications. Since the peptides are not orally
active, their role in the treatment of hypertension is uncertain
at this point. Their value as diagnostic tools has been
established. For example, the use of saralasin in the recogni-
tion of angiotensinogenic hypertension in man has been demonstrated (<u>103</u>). Perhaps of greater value will be the role of these
compounds and peptides still to come in defining the importance
of the renin-angiotensin system in the etiology of hypertension
and the control of blood pressure.

References Cited

1. "Physicians Desk Reference", 29th Ed., p. 687, Medical Economics Co., Oradell, N.J. (1975)
2. Druey, J. and Marxer, A., J. Med. Pharm. Chem. (1959) 1, 1.
3. Druey, J. and Tripod, J., "Antihypertensive Agents", pp. 223-262, ed. E. Schlittler, Academic Press, New York (1967).
4. Gross, F., Druey, J. and Meier, R., Experientia (1950) 6, 19.
5. Walker, H., Wilson, S., Atkins, E., Garrett, H. and Richardson, A., J. Pharmacol. Exptl. Therap., (1951) 101, 368.
6. Baldoli, E., Sardi, A., Dezulian, V., Capellini, M. and Bianchi, G., Arzneim.-forsch.(1973) 23, 1591.
7. Carpi, C. and Dorigotti, L., Brit. J. Pharmacol. (1974) 52, 459P.
8. Akashi, A., Chiba, T. and Kasahara, A., Europ. J. Pharmacol. (1974) 29, 161.
9. Rubin, A., Roth, F., Winburg, M., Topliss, J., Sherlock, M., Sperber, N. and Black, J., Science (1961) 133, 2067.
10. Topliss, J., Sherlock, M., Reimann, H., Konzelman, L., Shapiro, E., Pettersen, B., Schneider, H. and Sperber, N., J. Med. Chem. (1963) 6, 122.
11. Raffa, L., Lilla, L. and Grana, E., Farmaco, Ed. Sci. (1965) 20, 647.
12. Raffa, L., DiBella, M., Ferrari, P., Rinaldi, M. and Ferrari, W., Farmaco, Ed. Sci. (1974) 29, 411.
13. Topliss, J. and Yudis, M., J. Med. Chem. (1972) 15, 394.
14. Hess, H.-J., Cronin, T. and Scriabine, A., J. Med. Chem. (1968) 11, 130.
15. Cronin, T. and Hess, H.-J., J. Med. Chem. (1968) 11, 136.
16. Scriabine, A., Constantine, J., Hess, H.-J. and McShane, W., Experientia (1968) 24, 1150.
17. For a recent survey, see "Prazosin-Evaluation of a new anti-hypertensive agent." Proc. of a Symposium held at the Centre Interprof. Geneva (8.3.74) - Amsterdam. Exerpta Med./New York, Elselvier (1974).
18. DeGuia, D., Mendlowitz, M., Russo, C., Vlachakis, N. and Antram, S., Curr. Ther. Res. (1973) 15, 339.
19. Zins, G., J. Pharmacol. Exptl. Therap. (1965) 150, 109.
20. Zins, G., Emmert, D. and Walk, R., J. Pharmacol. Exptl. Therap. (1968) 159, 194.
21. Pettinger, W. and Mitchell, H., New Eng. J. Med. (1973) 289 167; Clin. Pharmacol. Therap. (1973) 14, 143.
22. Bennett, C. and Wilburn, R., Clin. Res. (1974) 22, 262A.
23. Kincaid-Smith, P., Amer. J. Cardiol. (1973) 32, 575.
24. Chidsey, C., Clin. Sci. Molec. Med. (1973) 45 (Suppl. I) 171s.
25. Pettinger, W., Campbell, W. and Keeton, K., Circulation Res. (1973) 33, 82.

26. O'Malley, K., Velasco, M. and McNay, J., Clin. Res. (1973)
    21, 953.
27. Pettinger, W. and Keeton, K., Clin. Res. (1973) 21, 472.
28. Ryan, J. Jain, A. and McMahon, F., Curr. Therap. Res. (1975)
    17, 55.
29. Matta, R. and Wooten, G., Clin. Pharmacol. Ther. (1973) 14,
    (4-I) 54.
30. Hidaka, H., Nagasaka, A. and Takeda, A., J. Clin. Endocrinol.
    and Metabolism (1973) 37, 145.
31. Hidaka, H., Asano, T. and Takemoto, N., Mol. Pharmacol.
    (1973) 9, 172.
32. Ishii, Y., Fujii, Y. and Umezawa, H., Jap. J. Pharmacol.
    (1973) 23, Suppl., 53 (Abstr. 76).
33. Hidaka, H., Hara, F., Harada, N., Hashizume, Y. and Yano, M.,
    J. Pharmacol. Exptl. Therap. (1974) 191, 384
34. Hidaka, H., Hara, F., Harada, N. and Asano, M., Jap. J.
    Pharmacol. (1974) 24, (Suppl.) 25 (Abstr. 5).
35. Harada, N. Hashizume, Y. and Hidaka, H., Jap. J. Pharmacol.
    (1974) 24 (Suppl.) 77 (Abstr. 110).
36. Velasco, M., Gilbert, C., Rutledge, C. and McNay, J., Circu-
    lation (1974) 50 (III) 105, abstr. 412.
37. Velasco, M. and McNay, J., Clin. Pharmacol. Ther. (1974) 15,
    222.
38. Symchowicz., S. and Staub, M., J. Pharmacol. Exptl. Therap.
    (1974) 191, 324.
39. Loev, B., Ehrreich, S. and Tedeschi, R., J. Pharm. Pharma-
    col. (1972) 24, 917.
40. Vater, W., Kroneberg, G., Hoffmeister, F., Kaller, H.,
    Meng, K., Oberdorf, A., Puls, W., Schlossmann, K. and
    Stoepel, K., Arzneim.-forsch. (1972) 22, 1 and succeeding
    articles.
41. Loev, B., Goodman, M., Snader, K., Tedeschi, R. and Macko,
    E., J. Med. Chem. (1974) 17, 956.
42. Petta, J. and McLean, R., quoted in Walkenstein, S.,
    Intoccia, A., Flanagan, T., Hwang, B., Flint, D.,
    Weinstock, J., Villani, A., Blackburn, D. and Green, H.,
    J. Pharm. Sci. (1973) 62, 580.
43. Ryan, J., Blumenthal, H. and McMahon, F., Clin. Pharm. Ther.
    (1975) 17, 243.
44. Takenaka, F., Takeya, N., Ishihara, T., Inoue, S., Tsutsumi,
    E., Nakamura, R., Mitsufiyi, Y. and Sumie, M., Jap. J.
    Pharmacol. (1970) 20, 253.
45. Goetz, M., Grozinger, K. and Oliver, J., J. Med. Chem. (1973)
    16, 671.
46. "Physicians Desk Reference," 29th. Ed., pp. 708, 1380,
    Medical Economics Co., Oradell, N. J. (1975).
47. Majid, P., Meevan, M., Benaim, M., Sherma, B. and Taylor,
    S., Brit. Heart. J. (1974) 36, 588.

48. Constantine, J., McShane, W., Scriabine, A. and Hess, H.-J., "Hypertension: Mechanisms and Management." Section VI, "Recent Advances in Drug Therapy," p. 429, 26th Hahnemann Symposium, Ed. Onesti, G., Kim, K. and Moyer, J., Grune and Stratton, New York (1973).
49. Lewis, P., George, C. and Dollery C., Europ. J. Clin. Pharmacol. (1973) 6, 211.
50. White, C., Royds, R. and Turner, P., Postgrad. Med. J. (1974) 50, 729.
51. Archibald, J., Alps, B., Cavalla, J. and Jackson, J., J. Med. Chem. (1971) 14, 1054.
52. Archibald, J. and Benke, G., J. Med. Chem. (1974) 17, 736.
53. Archibald, J., Fairbrother, P. and Jackson, J., J. Med. Chem. (1974) 17, 739.
54. Dorigotti, L. and Glasser, A., Pharmacol. Res. Commun., (1972) 4, 151.
55. Farmer, J., Kennedy, I., Levy, G. and Marshall, R., Brit. J. Pharmacol. (1972) 45, 660.
56. Collier, J., Dawnay, N., Nachev, C. and Robinson, B., Brit. J. Pharmacol. (1972) 44, 286.
57. Richards, D., Woodings, E., Stephens, M. and Maconochie, J., Brit. J. Clin. Pharmacol. (1974) 1, 505.
58. Skinner, C., Gaddie, J. and Palmer, K., Br. Med. J. (1975) 2, (5962) 59.
59. "Physicians Desk Reference," 29th Ed., p. 1489, Medical Economics Co., Oradell, N.J. (1975).
60. Exley, K., Brit. J. Pharmacol. (1957) 12, 297.
61. Boura, A., Green, A., McCoubrey, A., Lawrence, D., Moulton, R. and Rosenheim, J., Lancet (1959) II, 17.
62. Maxwell, R., Ross, S. and Plummer, A., J. Pharmacol. Exptl. Therap. (1958) 123, 128.
63. Page, I. and Dustan, H., J.A.M.A. (1959) 170, 1265.
64. Mull, R. and Maxwell, R., "Antihypertensive Agents," pp. 115-149, ed. E. Schlittler, Academic Press, New York, (1967).
65. deHaen, P., Clin. Pharmacol. Ther. (1974) 16, (3-I), 413.
66. Hansson, L., Pascual, A. and Julius, S., Clin. Pharmacol. Therap. (1973) 14, 204.
67. Bolme, P., Corrodi, H. and Fuxe, K., Acta, Pharmacol. Toxicol. (1972) 31, (Suppl. I) 65.
68. Saini, R., Caputi, A. and Marmo, E., Farmaco, Ed. Prat. (1973) 28, 359.
69. McMahon, F. G., Cole, P., Boyles, P. and Vanov, S., Curr. Ther. Res. (1974) 16, 389.
70. Sternberg, J., Sannerstedt, R. and Werkö, L., Europ. J. Clin. Pharmacol. (1971) 3, 63.
71. Ellenbogen, L., Chan, P. and Cummings, J., Arch. Int. Pharmacodyn. (1974) 207, 170.
72. Gadekar, S., Nibi, S. and Cohen, E., J. Med. Chem. 11, 811 (1968).

73. Matier, W., Owens, D., Comer, W., Deitchmann, D., Ferguson, H., Seidehamel, R. and Young, J., J. Med. Chem. (1973) 16, 901.
74. Perhach, J., Gomoll, A., Ferguson, H. and McKinney, G., Fed. Proc. (1974) 33, 485, Abstr. 1551.
75. Deitchmann, D. and Gomoll, A., Fed. Proc. (1974) 33, 485 Abstr. 1552.
76. Deitchmann, D., Gomoll, A., Snyder, R., and Preston, J., Arch. Int. Pharmacodyn. (1974) 210, 268.
77. Engelman, K., Horwitz, D., Jequier, E. and Sjoerdsma, A., J. Clin. Invest. (1968) 47, 577.
78. Engelman, K. and Sjoerdsma, A., Circulation Res. (1966) 18/19, Suppl. I, 104.
79. Day, M. and Rand, M., J. Pharm. Pharmacol. (1963) 15, 221.
80. Day, M. and Rand, M., Brit. J. Pharmacol. (1964) 22, 72.
81. Horwitz, D. and Sjoerdsma, A., Life Sci. (1964) 3, 41.
82. Holtmeier, H., vonKlein-Wisenberg, A. and Marongiu, F., Deutsche Med. Wochen. (1966) 91, 198.
83. Crout, J., Johnston, R., Webb, W. and Shore, P., Clin. Res. (1965) 13, 204.
84. Rangno, R., Kaufman, J., Cavanaugh, J., Island, D., Watson, J. and Oates, J., J. Clin. Invest. (1973) 52, 952.
85. Saari, W., Raab, A., Staas, W., Torchiana, M., Porter, C. and Stone, C., J. Med. Chem. (1970) 13, 1057.
86. Torchiana, M., Porter, C., Stone, C., Watson, L., Scriabine, A. and Hanson, H., Biochem. Pharmacol. (1971) 20, 1537.
87. Merrifield, R., J. Am. Chem. Soc. (1963) 85, 2149.
88. Bumpus, F., Sen, S., Smeby, R., Sweet, C., Ferrario, C. and Khosla, M., Circulation Res. (1973) 32/33 (Suppl.I) I-150.
89. Khosla, M., Hall, M., Smeby, R. and Bumpus, F., J. Med. Chem. (1974) 17, 431.
90. Park, W., Choi, C., Rioux, F. and Regoli, D., Can. J. Biochem. (1974) 52, 113.
91. Paiva, T., Goissis, G., Juliano, L., Miyamoto, M. and Paiva, A., J. Med. Chem. (1974) 17, 238.
92. Jorgensen, E., Kiraly-Olah, I., Lee, T. and Windridge, G., J. Med. Chem. (1974) 17, 323.
93. Khosla, M., Hall, M., Smeby, R. and Bumpus, F., J. Med. Chem. (1974) 17, 1156.
94. Sen, S., Smeby, R. and Bumpus, F., Proc. Soc. Exp. Biol. Med. (1974) 147, 847.
95. Pena, C., Stewart, J. and Goodfriend, T., Life Sci. (1974) 14, 1331.
96. Wissmann, H., Schoelkens, B., Lindner, E. and Geiger, R., Hoppe-Seylers Z. Physiol. Chem. (1974) 355, 1083.
97. Pals, D., Masucci, F., Denning, G., Sipos, F. and Fessler, D., Circulation Res. (1971) 29, 673.

98. Brunner, H., Gavras, H., Laragh, J. and Keenan, R., Lancet (1973) II, 1045.
99. Ondetti, M., Williams, N., Sabo, E., Pluscec, J., Weaver, E. and Kocy, O., Biochemistry (1971) 10, 4033.
100. Cushman, D., Pluscec, J., Williams, N., Weaver, E., Sabo, E., Kocy, O., Cheung, H. and Ondetti, M., Experientia (1973) 29, 1032.
101. Black, W., Shenouda, A., Johnson, J., Share, L., Shade, R., Friedman, B., Acchiardo, S., Vukovich, R., Hatch, F. and Muirhead, E., Clin. Res. (1974) 22, 263A.
102. Gavras, H., Brunner, H., Laragh, J., Sealey, J., Gavras, I. and Vukovich, R., New Engl. J. Med. (1974) 291, 817.
103. Anderson, G., Freiberg, J., Dalakos, T. and Streeten, D., Clin. Res. (1974) 22, 257A.

4

Antihypertensive Agents as Seen by the Clinician

GADDO ONESTI

Division of Nephrology and Hypertension, Hahnemann Medical College and Hospital, Philadelphia, Pa. 19102

It is now well accepted that sustained elevation of blood pressure for an adequate period of time in itself results in significant vascular damage throughout the body(1,2). It is also well recognized that lowering of the blood pressure with pharmacologic agents is effective in reducing morbidity and mortality not only in patients with malignant and severe hypertension(3), but also in patients with moderately severe and mild blood pressure elevation(4). Particularly, the survey by the Veterans Administration Hospital, reported in 1970, has provided final demonstration that antihypertensive therapy is capable of tangibly lowering the incidence of death and of adverse morbid events, even in patients with diastolic hypertensions between 90 and 114 mm Hg. (5).

Clearly, the ideal antihypertensive drug will be one which neutralizes a specific etiological factor responsible for the disease. Unfortunately, a specific etiology has not been found for the overwhelming number of hypertensive states in man. It is also becoming apparent that numerous factors regulate the blood pressure and that, therefore, numerous variables may be deranged in hypertension(6). Thus, an empirical approach is still necessary in the treatment of the hypertensive patients.

With the increasing number of pharmacologic agents, however, and with the acceptance of the concept of drug combination for effective therapy(7), the physician may select the most appropriate drug (or combination) for the individual clinical situation.

Deranged Circulatory Homeostasis in Hypertension

It is estimated that approximately 90% of the patients with blood pressure elevation are affected by essential hypertension, which is by definition, hypertension of unknown etiology. Although the mechanisms responsible for essential hypertension remain obscure, extensive hemodynamic studies have now revealed the precise derangements of the systemic hemodynamics of these patients(8).

The generally accepted equation describing the hemodynamic factors regulating blood pressure may be expressed in the form BP = CO x TPR; where BP is the mean arterial pressure, CO the cardiac output, and TPR the total peripheral resistance. Using this simplified equation, it may be concluded that high blood pressure may result from a high cardiac output, a high total peripheral resistance, or a combination of the two.

It is now apparent that young essential hypertension patients, in the early stage of the disease, have blood pressure elevations associated with high cardiac output and a normal peripheral resistance at rest. The high cardiac output is due to a high heart rate and normal stroke volume. It could, therefore, be concluded that a high cardiac output with high heart rate might be involved in the production of high blood pressure in young patients with essential hypertension(8). Even at this stage, however, a relative elevation of total peripheral resistance is demonstrable during exercise. We should, therefore, conclude that both the heart pump and the peripheral vessels are involved at the beginning of the hypertensive disease(8).

With advancing age, the patient with essential hypertension progressively changes his hemodynamic pattern into one of normal cardiac output with increased peripheral arteriolar constriction and, finally, later in the natural course of the disease into one of lower cardiac output and further increase in peripheral vascular resistance(8).

Factors which have been considered responsible for this hemodynamic alteration are: heredity, salt and water, the adrenergic nervous system and the renin-angiotensin system.

The Ideal Antihypertensive Agent

If a totally rational attack based on the etiology is impossible, the empirical approach is necessary at this time.

An ideal antihypertensive agent should have the following characteristics:
1) orally active
2) sufficiently prolonged duration of action
3) effective in supine and standing positions, at rest and during exercise
4) normalize the hemodynamic derangements
5) free from adverse side reactions

Peripheral Vasodilators

If the hemodynamic defect in essential hypertension is peripheral arteriolar vasoconstriction with increased total peripheral vascular resistance, peripheral vasodilators would appear an ideal therapeutic approach.

Indeed, hydralazine has been effectively used for the management of hypertension for over 20 years. The decrease in

blood pressure produced by peripheral vasodilatation results in
significant stimulation of the baroreceptors. The baroreceptor
mechanism is, therefore, activated and increased adrenergic discharge from the vasomotor centers reaches the heart and the peripheral vessels. This cardiovascular reflex results in a sharp
increase in cardiac output and heart rate. Thus, although
hydralazine can decrease total peripheral resistance by 50-60%,
its effect on blood pressure is much less because of the compen-
satory increase in cardiac output(9).

Hydralazine is equally effective in the supine and standing
positions. The cardiovascular reflexes are intact and no postural
hypotension is seen. However, the reflex tachycardia and increase
in cardiac output (Figure 1) severely limit the clinical use of
this drug. Tachycardia is almost invariably associated with the
subjective complaints of severe palpitations (Figure 1).

Together with the increase in cardiac output, renal blood
flow is also increased with a significant decrease in renal vascular resistance(10).

Because of their reflex cardiac effect, vasodilators, if
used alone in the treatment of hypertension, have not been a successful therapeutic tool. However, the reflex tachycardia and increase in cardiac output can be effectively blocked by the therapeutic association with a sympathetic blocker: guanethidine,
reserpine, methyldopa, or clonidine. More specifically, blockade
of the cardiac beta-adrenergic receptors will also prevent the
cardiac response to hydralazine. Thus, the therapeutic combination of hydralazine and propranolol can be successfully employed
for effective blood pressure reduction(11).

Diuretic Agents

Dietary salt restriction was one of the first successful
therapeutic maneuvers for the reduction of blood pressure. During
the past two decades, a variety of pharmacologic agents have been
developed which promote diuresis by interfering with the tubular
reabsorption of sodium. Although diuretic agents differ significantly in chemical structure and in their mechanism of action on
the renal tubule, they all have in common the ability to decrease
blood pressure.

Despite their successful use for at least 20 years, the
mechanisms by which they lower the blood pressure remain uncertain. Theories to explain the antihypertensive effectiveness
of the diuretic agents have included: a) alteration of sodium
and water content on arterial smooth muscle, b) the induction of
a decreased vascular response to catecholamines, c) a decrease in
blood volume and total extracellular fluid volume, and d) a direct
vasodilator action independent from the diuretic effect(12).

From a hemodynamic standpoint, chlorothiazide has been shown
to exert a diphasic action on systemic hemodynamics: first, the
decrease in blood pressure is associated with a decrease in blood

volume and a decrease in cardiac output. Later, after more prolonged administration, blood volume and cardiac output return to
pretreatment levels, while total peripheral resistance shows a
significant decrease. This hemodynamic event demonstrates that
the long term effects of the thiazide diuretics (and possibly
non-thiazide diuretics) is indeed vasodilatation(13,14).

The blood pressure reduction by the diuretic agents occurs
equally in supine, sitting and standing positions, at rest and
during exercise. There is no orthostatic hypotension(13,14).

The most important side effects of the thiazide diuretics,
chlorthalidone, furosemide, ethacrynic acid and metolazone are:
potassium losses with resultant hypokalemia, and hyperuricemia.
Hyperuricemia may result in acute attacks of gouty arthritis in
individuals with a gouty diathesis.

The aldosterone antagonist, spironolactone, has been successfully used for the treatment of hypertension. Its natriuretic
effect is associated with potassium retention. Specificity of
spironolactone in certain types of hypertension had been suggested, but subsequently denied in well controlled studies(15,16).

Triamterene is also a diuretic with distal tubule action and
potassium retaining properties. It is not generally used alone
as an antihypertensive agent.

In order to correct potassium losses and the consequent diu-
retic-induced hypokalemia, spironolactone or triamterene can be
successfully combined with the thiazide, metolazone, chlorthalidone, furosemide or ethacrynic acid.

It is now becoming apparent that a single daily dose (rather
than 2-3 doses per day) significantly enhances patient compliance
and, therefore, effectiveness of treatment. For this reason, the
long-acting diuretics which can be administered once a day offer
an important advantage: chlorthalidone, metolazone, trichlor-
methiazide can be administered once a day with a 24 hour natriuretic effect.

Furosemide and ethacrynic acid preserve glomerular filtration rate and are, therefore, the diuretic agents of choice in
hypertensive patients with impairment of kidney function(17,18,
19). Spironolactone may induce painful gynecomastia and impo-
tence in the male, and menstrual irregularities in the female.
For this reason, spironolactone is not the diuretic of choice for
long-term treatment of hypertension. Its major use appears to be
in combination with other diuretics for the purpose of maintaining
potassium balance.

Because of their capability of lowering the blood pressure
regardless of body position, of their overall excellent acceptance by the patients and because of their favorable hemodynamic
effects, the diuretic agents remain the most important contribu-
tion to antihypertensive therapy.

Equally important as their ability to lower blood pressure
when used alone is the potentiation of all other antihypertensive
drugs(7). The most commonly accepted explanation for this

potentiation is that when non-diuretic antihypertensive agents
lower the blood pressure, the kidney responds to the decreased
perfusion pressure with retention of sodium chloride and water.
This leads to expansion of plasma and extracellular fluid volume,
thus attenuating or abolishing the original decrease in blood
pressure. Concomitant administration of a diuretic is, therefore,
necessary when other antihypertensive drugs are given.

Thus, diuretics, alone or in combination with other anti-
hypertensive agents, represent the cornerstone of our antihypertensive armamentarium.

Inhibitors of Peripheral Sympathetic Systems

Historically, the first effective pharmacologic agents for
lowering the blood pressure were the ganglionic blockers. At the
level of the ganglia, these compounds block both sympathetic and
parasympathetic transmission. The decrease in parasympathetic
function is responsible for urinary retention, for the failure to
develop an erection in the male patient and for the paralytic
ileus.

The inhibition of sympathetic tone to the venous system
(capacitance vessels) results in increased pooling of blood in
the venous vascular bed with consequent decreased venous return
to the heart and decreased cardiac output. This phenomenon is
more pronounced in upright positions because of the effect of
gravity. The hemodynamic effects of ganglionic blockers include:
decreases in cardiac output, renal blood flow, cerebral blood
flow and orthostatic hypotension(20,21).

A significant advance in pharmacology was achieved with the
introduction of guanethidine. Guanethidine may be considered the
prototype of sympathetic inhibitors acting at the level of the
post-ganglionic sympathetic nerve ending. The drug depletes the
neurotransmitter (norepinephrine at this site) and prevents neuro-
humoral transmission. The absence of parasympathetic blockade
represented a significant improvement over the ganglionic blockers.
The hemodynamic effects of guanethidine, however, are determined
by the decrease in sympathetic tone to the capacitance vessels and
to the arterioles as well. Similar to that described for the
ganglionic blockers, guanethidine results in decreases in cardiac
output, (Figure 2), renal blood flow, glomerular filtration rate
(Figure 3), and cerebral blood flow(9). Reduced cerebral blood
flow manifests itself clinically by light-headedness. Decreased
perfusion of the skeletal muscles results in fatigability. Orthostatic hypotension is prominent. Thus, from a hemodynamic standpoint, the circulatory defect of essential hypertension in man is
certainly not corrected by this agent.

It is now becoming apparent that peripheral inhibition of
sympathetic transmission, although effective in lowering blood
pressure, does not restore circulatory homeostasis in the hypertensive patient, and in the light of recent progress in the

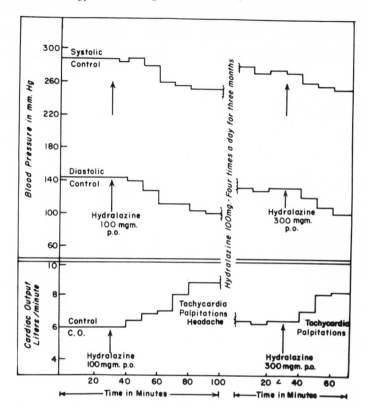

Figure 1.   Cardiac output and blood pressure response in patient
with hypertension

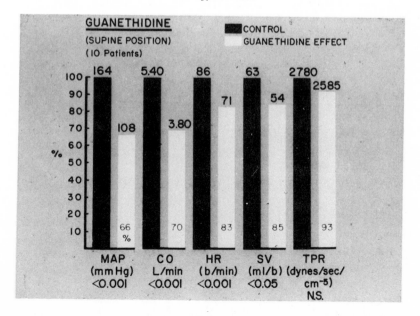

Figure 2.

pharmacotherapy of hypertension must be considered of only historical importance.

The Rauwolfia alkaloids lower the blood pressure through various mechanisms. The antihypertensive effect is probably due primarily to the depletion of norepinephrine in the postganglionic nerve endings. There is also an important effect on the brain biogenic amines. When administered orally for long-term therapy of hypertension, these compounds exert only a modest antihypertensive effect. Their effectiveness, however, may be enhanced by the concomitant administration of a diuretic(7). Because of the overall selective sympathetic inhibition, these drugs may result in overriding manifestations of predominant parasympathetic effects. Thus, increased gastric secretion, peptic ulcer, increased intestinal motility, nasal arteriolar dilatation with nasal stuffiness, are common side effects. In addition, because of the depletion of brain amines and serotonin, behavioral changes are to be expected. Although severe mental depression is relatively rare, subtle subclinical depression is frequent. This may be manifested by lack of energy, insomnia, and inefficiency in job performance. These subtle behavioral effects of the Rauwolfia compounds should limit their widespread use when other pharmacologic agents are available.

Antihypertensive Agents Acting on the Vasomotor Centers

Methyldopa was developed in order to obtain an inhibitor of the dopa-decarboxylase enzyme system, thus preventing the step dopa to dopamine in the biosynthesis of norepinephrine. The decreased availability of norepinephrine was expected to decrease blood pressure. Indeed, dopa-decarboxylase inhibition and antihypertensive action were recognized. It soon became apparent, however, that the biochemical and cardiovascular effects of methyldopa were unrelated. Subsequently, it was demonstrated that conversion of methyldopa into alpha-methylnorepinephrine was essential for achieving blood pressure reduction. This finding generated the "false neurotransmitter theory". According to this interpretation, alpha-methylnorepinephrine, generated by metabolism of methyldopa, displaced the true neurotransmitter norepinephrine. Although this seems to be an interesting mechanism, the explanation now is considered incomplete.

In 1967, Henning and Van Zwieten provided conclusive evidence that the most important effect of methyldopa is on the vasomotor centers in the central nervous system(22). This central effect results in a decrease in sympathetic tone to the periphery.

In addition, there is now good evidence indicating that methyldopa effectively suppresses the release of renin by the kidney(23,24). This effect may contribute to the antihypertensive efficacy of the drug in some hypertensive states in which the renin-angiotensin system plays a pathophysiologic role. Thus, it may be concluded that a) methyldopa lowers the blood pressure

primarily by action on the vasomotor centers resulting in decreased sympathetic outflow; b) peripheral sympathetic modulation
through the "false neurotransmitter" mechanism may add to the
cardiovascular effect of the drug(25); c) the inhibition of renin
release may contribute to the effectiveness of methyldopa in certain clinical situations.

The hemodynamic effects of methyldopa in patients with essential hypertension differ significantly from those of the peripheral sympathetic inhibitors. Administration of methyldopa
results in a decrease in blood pressure, a preservation of cardiac
output and a significant decrease in total peripheral vascular
resistance(26,27) (Figure 4). At the same time, cerebral vascular
resistance is decreased with a well maintained cerebral blood flow
(28). In addition, while blood pressure is decreased, renal blood
flow remains unchanged and renal vascular resistance is decreased
(26) (Figure 5). Thus, the hemodynamic effects of methyldopa
approach the ideal restoration of circulatory homeostasis. A
predominantly orthostatic antihypertensive effect is, however,
present. This is presumably due to the peripheral sympathetic
inhibition ("false neurotransmitter") and is significantly less
apparent than with ganglionic blockers or guanethidine.

Methyldopa has been used for approximately 15 years. The
most common side effects are somnolence, hemolytic anemia (rare),
appearance of a direct Coombs test (frequent), methyldopa fever
and hepatotoxicity (rare).

Another antihypertensive agent with action on the vasomotor
centers is clonidine. Kobinger and co-workers demonstrated in
the experimental animal that clonidine lowers the blood pressure
by a direct effect on the vasomotor centers(29). This effect results in a centrally mediated decrease in sympathetic discharge
while vagal tone is increased(30,31). There is no inhibition of
sympathetic neurotransmission at the level of the ganglion nor at
post-ganglionic sites. The hemodynamic effect of this central
action is distributed between cardiac output, heart rate, and peripheral vascular resistance. There is a predictable decrease in
heart rate and cardiac output. The total peripheral resistance
effect is evident in the standing position (Figure 6). Renal
blood flow is maintained with a consistent decrease in renal
vascular resistance(32) (Figure 7). Also, muscle blood flow is
preserved. After acute administration of clonidine, the blood
pressure reduction is more marked in the standing position. After
prolonged administration, however, there is no detectable difference between supine and upright blood pressure(32). Clinically, no orthostatic hypotension is reported. Thus, while sympathetic outflow from the vasomotor center is decreased by clonidine, central integration of cardiovascular reflexes mediated by
the baroreceptors appears to be preserved.

Both in the experimental animal and in patients, administration of clonidine suppresses renin release by the kidney(32)
(Figure 8). These observations suggest the possibility that this

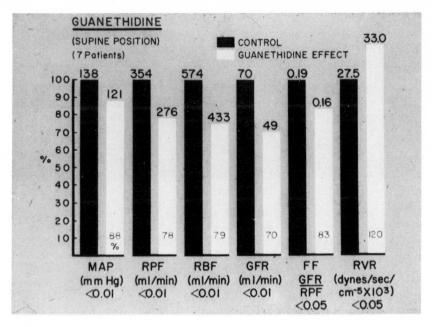

Figure 3.

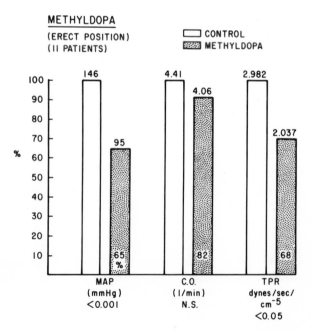

Figure 4.

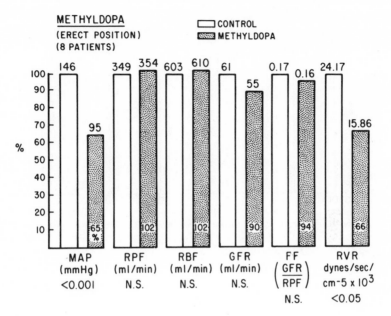

Figure 5.

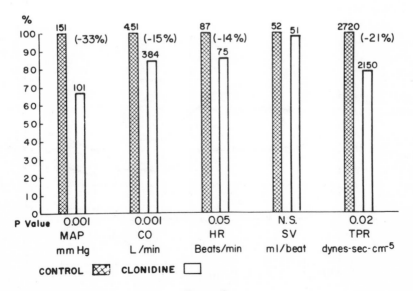

Figure 6.

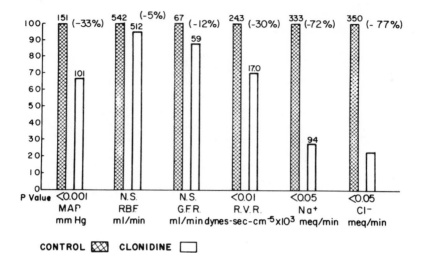

Figure 7.

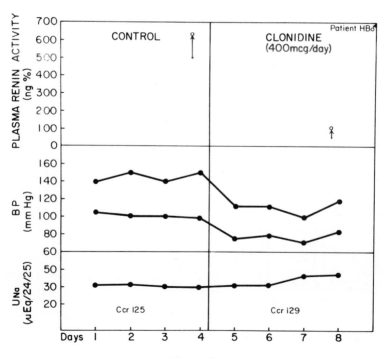

Figure 8.

effect may contribute to the antihypertensive effectiveness of
the drug in hypertensive states in which the renin-angiotensin
system plays a pathophysiologic role.

Clinically, clonidine has shown great versatility: effective in mild, moderate and severe hypertension. The major side
effects are drowsiness and dry mouth. Clonidine can be effectively used in combination with a diuretic(32). In addition, a
vasodilator (hydralazine) can be usefully added. The brady-
cardiac effect of clonidine prevents the reflex tachycardia induced by the vasodilator.

In general, the introduction of antihypertensive agents
acting on the vasomotor center in the brain appears to be a major
advance in the treatment of hypertension. The well balanced
hemodynamic effect is far superior to what is observed with inhibition of sympathetic transmission at peripheral sites. Orthostatic hypotension is no longer a problem. It is predicted that
pharmacologic progress in this line of compounds will make further contributions to our antihypertensive armamentarium.

Literature Cited

1. Dublin, L.J., Lotka, A.J. and Spiegelman, M., "Length of
   Life, a Study of the Life Table", Ronald Press, Ed. 2,
   New York, (1949).
2. Bechgaard, P., Kopp, H. and Nielsen, J., Acta Med. Scand.,
   (1955), 309, 175.
3. Moyer, J.H., Heider, C., Pevey, K. and Ford, R.V., Amer. J.
   Med., (1958), 24, 177.
4. Veterans Administration Cooperative Study Group on Antihypertensive Agents: Effects of treatment on morbidity in hypertension: I. Results in patients with diastolic blood pres-
   sures averaging 115 through 129 mm Hg., J.A.M.A., (1967),
   202, 1028.
5. Veterans Administration of Cooperative Study Group on Anti-
   hypertensive Agents: Effects of treatment on morbidity in
   hypertension. II. Results in patients with diastolic blood
   pressure averaging 90 through 114 mm Hg., J.A.M.A., (1970),
   213, 1143.
6. Guyton, A.C., Coleman, T.G. and Granger, H.J., Ann. Rev.
   Physiol., (1972), 34, 13.
7. Brest, A.N., "Antihypertensive Therapy", Springer-Verlag,
   302, F. Gross, Editor, New York, (1966).
8. Lund-Johansen, P., Acta. Med. Scand., (1967), Suppl. 482,
   181, 1.
9. Onesti, G., Kwan, E.K., Swartz, C. and Moyer, J.H., "Hypertension: Mechanisms and Management", Grune and Stratton, 227,
   New York and London, (1973).
10. Vanderkolk, K., Dontas, A.S. and Hoobler, S.W., Am. Heart J.,
    (1954), 48, 95.
11. Gottlieb, T.B., Katz, F.H., Chidsey, C.A., Circulation,

(1972), 45, 571.

12. Tarazi, R., "Hypertension: Mechanisms and Management", Grune
     and Stratton, 251, New York and London, (1973).
13. Freis, E.D., "Essential Hypertension", Springer-Verlag, 179,
     Berlin, (1960).
14. Villarreal, H., Exaire, J.E., Revollo, A. and Soni, J., Cir-
     culation, (1962), 26, 405.
15. Johnston, L.C. and Greible, H.G., Arch. Intern. Med., (1967),
     119, 225.
16. Crane, M.G. and Harris, J.J., Am. J. Med. Sci., (1970), 260,
     311.
17. Davidov, M., Kakaviatos, N. and Finnerty, F.A., Jr., Circu-
     lation, (1967), 36, 125.
18. Birtch, A.G., Zakheim, R.M., Jones, L.G. and Barger, A.C.,
     Circ. Res., (1967), 21, 869.
19. Nash, H.L., Fitz, A.E., Wilson, W., Kirkendall, W.M. and
     Kioschos, J.M., Am. Heart J., (1966), 71, 153.
20. Freis, E.D., Rose, J.D., Partenope, E.A., Higgins, T.F.,
     Kelley, R.T., Schnaper, H.W. and Johnson, R.D., J. Clin.
     Invest., (1953), 32, 1285.
21. Trapold, J.H., Circ. Res., (1957), 5, 444.
22. Henning, M. and van Zwieten, P.A., J. Pharm. Pharmacol.,
     (1967), 19, 403.
23. Mohammed, S., Fasola, A.F., Privitera, P.J., Lipicky, R.J.,
     Martz, B.L. and Gaffney, T.E., Circ. Res., (1969), 25, 543.
24. Halushka, P.V., Keiser, H.R., Circ. Res., (1974), 35, 458.
25. Henning, M., Acta. Physiol. Scand., (1969a), Suppl. 322, 1.
26. Onesti, G., Brest, A.N., Novack, P., Kasparian, H., Moyer,
     J.H., Amer. Heart J., (1964), 67, 32.
27. Sannerstedt, R., Bojs, G., Varnauskas, E. and Werko, L.,
     Acta. Med. Scand., (1963), 174, 53.
28. Meyer, J.S., Sawada, T., Kitamura, A. and Toyoda, M.,
     Neurology (Minneap.), (1968), 18, 772.
29. Kobinger, W. and Walland, A., Eur. J. Pharmacol., (1967), 2,
     155.
30. Schmitt, H., Schmitt, H., Boissier, J.R., Giudicelli, J.F.,
     Eur. J. Pharmacol., (1967), 2, 147.
31. Kobinger, W. and Walland, A., Eur. J. Pharmacol., (1972), 19,
     203.
32. Onesti, G., Schwartz, A.B., Kim, K.E., Paz-Martinez, V. and
     Swartz, C., Circ. Res., (1971), Suppl. 2, 28, 53.

INDEX